AF544823

AIDS - HIV

A PRESCRIPTION FOR SURVIVAL

A Self Help Book

Hyperthermia, Autoimmune Therapy, and Drugs.
(Hyperthermia and The Water with Life, Volume I)

T. R. Shantha, M.D.(Cal), Ph.D.(USA)
Georgia Baptist Medical Center,
300 Boulevard NE, Atlanta, Ga 30312
Visiting Professor, JJM Medical College

Previously: Assistant surgeon, Mysore Medical Service; Associate Professor in the Departments of Anatomy, Ophthalmology, and Anesthesiology, Emory University School of Medicine; Director, Neurohistochemistry, Yerkes Regional Primate Research Center; Associate Chairman, Dept. of Anesthesiology, Georgia Baptist Medical Center; Staff member, Columbus Medical Center.

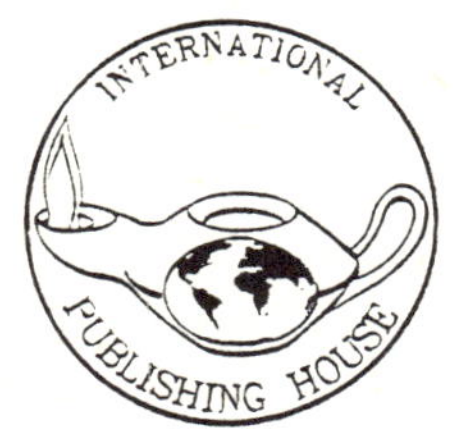

International Publishing House
Suite B, 1657 Kanawha Drive
Stone Mountain, GA 30087, U.S.A.
Telephone: 404/496-1482
1-800-767-CURE(2873)

Library of Congress catalog-in-publication data

Due to budget cuts the Library of Congress has not issued a catalog-in-publication data.

Shantha, T. R.

AIDS-HIV: A prescription for Survival.
(With Hyperthermia, Autoimmune Therapy, and drugs. Hyperthermia and The Water with Life:Volume I.)
By Dr.T.R. Shantha

ISBN 1-879144-01-8
EAN 9 781879 144019

1. How to cure or curtail AIDS and eliminate HIV infection. 1st Title
2. Hyperthermia, Autoimmune Urine Therapy, and Drugs for AIDS. 2nd Title
3. Cure for Incurable Diseases. 3rd Title

Published by:
International Publishing House
Suite B, 1657 Kanawha Drive
Stone Mountain, Georgia 30087, U.S.A.
Telephone 404/496-1482
1-800-767-CURE (2873)

Printed in U.S.A.
Cover Design by Patton H. McGinley, Jr.

DEDICATION

This book is dedicated to my late mother, Totada Gowramma, and father, T. Ramaiah; to my wife Victoria Kay T. Shantha and children (Devendra T., Usha T., Anand T., Jessica Gowramma T., Erica Maya T., and Lauren Asha Ruth T. Shantha), who gave me time and support during my personal experiments with Hyperthermia and Autoimmune Urine Therapy, acted as guinea pigs and helped in preparation of this manuscript.

DISCLAIMER

The contents of this book do not reflect the opinion or the method of treatment of the Georgia Baptist Medical Center, its commission members, staff members, Medical Center Anesthesia Associates, or any other members associated with our hospital or group. The contents of this book reflect the scientific ideas and research thoughts of the author and no one else. The author, the hospital and the departments he is associated with are not legally or otherwise responsible for any complications or adverse reactions arising due to the use of treatment recommended in this book.

DISTRIBUTED BY

J. A. Majors Co., 3770 A Zip Industrial Blvd.,
Atlanta, Georgia 30354, U.S.A.
(404) 768-4956, 1-800-241-6551

Individual readers, retailers, and distributors can order the books from the publishers. Bulk order discounts are available.

International Publishing House
Suite B, 1657 Kanawha Drive
Stone Mountain, GA 30087, U.S.A.
Telephone: 404/496-1482,
1-800-767-CURE (2873)

A SYMBOL OF EXCELLENCE

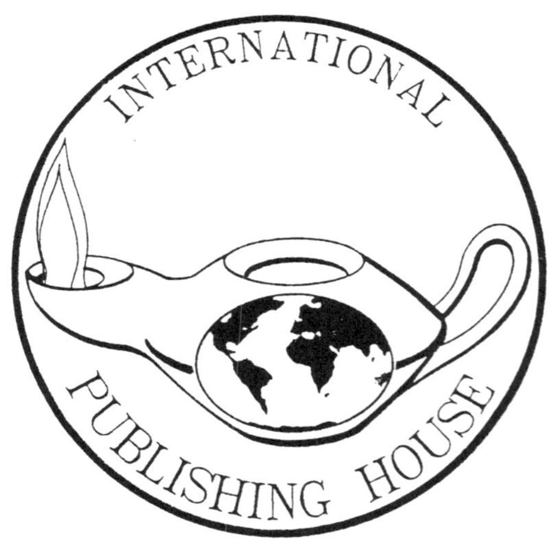

TABLE OF CONTENTS

CHAPTER 1

HYPERTHERMIA TREATMENT FOR AIDS, HIV POSITIVE, AND OTHER INCURABLE ACUTE AND CHRONIC DISEASES

By Using, Radiant heat, Dry Sauna, Hot Water And Other Methods

The elements will be destroyed by fire.

2 Peter 3:10

. . . nothing is hidden from its heat.

Psalms 19:6

The two of them were thrown alive into the fiery lake of burning sulfur.

Revelations 19:20

The greatest potential for local, regional or whole body hyperthermia comes from it's use as an adjunct to other methods of treatments.

T. R. Shantha

History

Increasing the body temperature to treat many kinds of disease has been in vogue throughout history. In Greece, Hippocrates introduced an Egyptian hot bath custom to treat various diseases. In Rome, Celsus treated joint pains, hysteria, dropsy, convulsions and kidney diseases with sweating baths. In the 17th century, the Japanese treated syphilis, arthritis, and gout by balneotherapy (treatment by baths).

Fever is often perceived as the harbinger of serious disease. As a matter of fact, it is often the body's method of fighting diseases. Hyperthermia is another term used to raise the body temperature by artificial methods. Whole body hyperthermia, alone or combined with radiation and chemotherapy is still being experimented in various research centers for treating advanced cancers. Elevated body temperature is beneficial to the cancer patient and originated nearly 125 years ago with reports of permanent cure or prolonged remission of cancers in patients who recovered from high fever after infection (Busch W: Akad Wis Nat Lng Wirtsch Vortr 23 , 28, 1866). Dr. Spranck in 1892 and Dr. W. B. Coley an orthopedic surgeon in 1893 published reports of curing bone sarcomas and cancers by inducing hyperthermia by injection of mixture of Erysipelas (Streptococcal) bacterial products (Annales de L'institut Pasteur 1892, Am J Med Sci 105, 487-511, 1893). In 1935, Warren Stafford treated 32 cases of advanced cancers by heating up to 42° for as long as 21 hours. This method of therapy was rejuvenated by a Scottish anesthesiologist, Dr. R. T. Pettigrew, in 1974. He induced hyperthermia by immersing the body in hot wax and inhalation of heated anesthetic gases (Br J Surg 61:727-730, 1974, Br Med J 4:679-682, 1974).

Background

In 1981, we (Dr. William Logan and our anesthesiology group) treated some advanced cancer patients with hyperthermia. I was involved in maintaining the patient's life support system and administering general anesthesia during hyperthermia. Anesthesiologists play a major role in total body hyperthermia using extracorporeal method (Fig.1). I had a long discussion with Dr. H. Logan about hyperthermia in the Georgia Baptist Medical Center's doctors lobby, on February 19, 1990. He induced hyperthermia using the extracorporeal method on an AIDS patient on February 20, 1990. I requested him to include autoimmune urine therapy (AUT) and hyperthermia treatment as I recommend in this book to achieve a cure. At that meeting, I told him, that I discussed the effects of hyperthermia and it's possible benefits in AIDS when combined with autoimmune therapy in my forthcoming book on AIDS.

Emory University held the eleventh annual Dr. Evan L. Fredrickson research lecture in the Medical Association of Georgia building on 22nd of June 1990. It was given by the distinguished professor Dr. John W. Severinghaus from the University of California at San Francisco, on the history of blood gas analysis and development of oxygen measuring devices. At that meeting the anesthesiologist from the Atlanta hospital where the hyperthermia was used on the first AIDS patient told me that they use the protocol developed by me in 1981 for cancer hyperthermia. This protocol was given to them by Dr. Logan. I was very glad that strict critical care and anesthesia guidelines are followed as set forth by me in that monograph.

I wrote about the possible benefits of hyperthermia in the treatment of AIDS when I started writing this book almost three years ago, even before it was tried in an Atlanta hospital. Based on what we know about the AIDS virus, I doubt very much that hyperthermia alone will eliminate HIV. I do believe that it should be used as an adjunct therapy. AIDS virus is incorporated into genetic material, and it is difficult or impossible to kill them at 108° F. The claim of cure by hyperthermia based on one case of AIDS is premature. It does help to cure or curtail Kaposi's sarcoma. I have a feeling that after some time the virus will multiply and disease will relapse unless the therapy is repeated and combined with other methods, as described in this chapter and chapter 9, 14, 18 and 19.

I believe that the extracorporeal method to induce hyperthermia is an invasive, expensive and life-threatening procedure. It needs general anesthesia, a vascular surgeon, a perfusionist, a host of paramedical people and intensive care. The whole body hyperthermia with such high temperature may not be needed to treat AIDS. There are other methods, such as radiant heating methods, available which are safer, less invasive and achieve the same goal. This field is for pure research scientists, not for the entrepreneur. Any physician performing this procedure without proper research background is using this method purely for publicity and financial gains.

One AIDS patient died in Mexico City undergoing extracorporeal method of hyperthermia in July 1990. According to the news media, the patient paid $50,000.00 for the treatment. There are excellent facilities and critical care available in this country than any place in the world. A trip to any foreign country for hyperthermia treatment can become a one-way trip.

Hundreds of articles are published and continued to be published on hyperthermia and its benefits in cancer. Now, the attention is focused on heating cancers locally instead of whole body hyperthermia. The whole body hyperthermia has not been investigated to treat other diseases. I believe that the whole body hyperthermia, autoimmune urine therapy, drugs, surgery, and radiation holds a place in treating diseases like AIDS, leprosy, tuberculosis, cancers, rabies, Alzheimer's, atherosclerotic disease of the blood vessels, skin diseases, autoimmune diseases, multiple sclerosis, addiction, microbial infections resistent to antibiotics, etc. Severe hyperthermia aggravates multiple sclerosis. Mild to moderate hyperthermia, along with AUT, should be tried in such cases.

There is a medical journal and a society devoted to hyperthermia (International Journal and Society of Hyperthermia). Radiologic Clinic of North America devoted its entire issue on hyperthermia (Volume 27, May 1989). The Massachusetts Institute of Technology has a division of hyperthermia center located at 77 Massachusetts Avenue, Room No. 17-434, Cambridge, Ma. 02139.

I have given all this information and some important references so that more research orientated physicians and patients themselves can make use of this therapy. If you cannot understand any material in this book and need to know more about it, please contact the publisher with postage paid, self-addressed envelope with $100.00 money order or credit card number. Read a couple of times, you will get the idea how to start hyperthermia program in your house setting with minimal equipment. **Many of the drugs and equipment I describe are needed only if you are undergoing severe hyperthermia for long periods of time. Don't be discouraged by reading this chapter and give up thinking this procedure is highly technical and cannot be accomplished.**

What is Hyperthermia?

Definition: Hyperthermia, fever, or hyperpyrexia is defined as an increase in temperature beyond that normally found in the body. This rise in temperature may be limited to local, regional or involve the whole body.

It also means treatment by artificially raising the body temperature. Hyperthermia can be induced by injection of malarial parasites or foreign proteins into the circulation, by immersing the body in hot wax, hot water or heated suits, by taking the blood by special tubing and heating the blood by special water heated coils and giving it back to the patient (extracorporeal heating), and by using radiant heat.

Humans are warm blooded (homoisothermic) compared to the col blooded fish, amphibians, and reptiles (poikilothermic). The normal body temperature is 98. 6°F (37° C). It can be within the range if it is above 1° or 2° below the value. Rectal temperature is always 0. 5 to 1. 0° F higher than oral temperature. For every centigrade increase in temperature, the basal energy expenditure increases by 12%. In most infections, the fever is the result of bacterial toxins and products affecting the heat regulating center in the brain. Dehydration, heat stroke, injury to the brain, extreme physical exercise, proteins and their products, etc., can also cause fever or hyperthermia. Certain families with genetic defect are prone to develop high fever under anesthesia or after strenuous exercise. It is called malignant hyperthermia. They will die if it is not recognized early and treated with the specific drug called Dantrolene.

Mechanism of Heat Transfer in Our Body

There are many ways by which the body exchanges head with external environment:

1. **Conduction:** Heat exchanges by transfer of thermal energy from atom to atom or molecule to molecule. Heat, like any other quantity, moves down a concentration gradient. Thus the body gains or loses heat by conduction only through direct contact with cooler or warmer substance including air, water, blankets, etc.

2. **Convection:** Here air or water next to the body is heated or cooled and moves away and is replaced by cool or warmer air and water.
3. **Radiation:** Heat is transferred by electromagnetic waves such as sun and special heaters.
4. **Evaporation:** When water evaporates from the body surfaces, such as skin and lungs, the heat required to drive the processes is absorbed from the surface, thereby by cooling it. You may not know that you lose more than 1/2 gallon (600 ml) water from lungs during breathing (expiration) by this process.

The adult human body has 2.5 million sweat glands and can produce 4 liters per hour sweat (9 lb of water). This will eliminate 1200 K cal from the body. Humidity in air plays a major role in our comfort or discomfort. Man can survive 266° F for 20 minutes or longer if the air is dry. Moist air at 115° F is difficult to breathe even a few minutes. Most of the claims of 10-20 pounds of weight loss during the early weeks of weight loss program by weight control centers is mostly due to fluid loss and not due to actual fat loss.

Effects of Hyperthermia

It is well established in laboratory as well as in several clinical studies that:

1. The primary effect of hyperthermia is direct thermal destruction of cancer cells, microbes, infected body cells, old cells, or in disease states. Temperatures above 42 degree centigrade kills healthy and unhealthy cells. Multiplying cells such as blood cells, cancer cells, HIV infected T4 lymphocytes, and other white blood cells are more sensitive to heat than healthy non-multiplying cells (Dickson JA: Cancer Chemotherapy Report 58:294-296, 1974).
2. Cancer cells are more sensitive to heat than normal cells. Likewise, AIDS infected cells are also sensitive to heat.
3. Heat potentiates the effects of radiation on both malignant and normal cells.
4. Hyperthermia is one of the most potent drug sensitizer we know. Heat synergistically interacts with a variety of antitumor

drugs. In the same fashion the microbe infected cells are also sensitized to drugs, antibodies, lymphokines, hormones, enzymes, and many known and unknown macromolecules. So hyperthermia should be combined with AUT with or without the specific drugs such as AZT, ddI and other drugs used in opportunistic infections in AIDS. As the AIDS virus is incorporated into the genetic material, I do not see how by raising the temperature to 108° F can get rid of all the infected cells.

5. Hyperthermia increases cell uptake and inhibits the repair mechanism in the damaged cells. This results in the cell's inability to pump drugs out from inside. This increases the concentration of drugs and antibodies within the afflicted cells and microbes resulting in their destruction. This synergetic action of hyperthermia may cure AIDS, leprosy, rabies, tuberculosis etc. when combined with AUT and drugs.
6. The cancer cells and HIV infected cells also develop reduction in oxygen dependent glucose breakdown and utilization (increased aerobic glycolysis), whereas normal cells do not show any such change with raise in body temperature. Hyperthermia sensitizes cancer cells to radiation and reduces the radiation dose by half required to kill cancer cells. AIDS virus, other microbes and infected cells are sensitized to antiviral drugs and antimicrobial such as AZT, ddI, PAS, Dapsone, INH, etc. Due to this change, even the small amount of drugs, antibodies, lymphokines, and interferon become effective. Surprisingly, it has been noted that the elevated oxygen level and increased oxygen delivery may antagonize the effect of hyperthermia.
7. Animal studies have shown that, when hyperthermia is applied locally to tumors, there is slow reabsorption of the dead cells which lead to potentiation of host immune response. This leads to subsequent destruction of metastatic tumors (Muckle DS, Dickson JA: Br J Cancer 27:307-315, 1974). In the same fashion, the urine rich in antigens during hyperthermia leads to development of immunity against the virus. It is like Dr. Fleck's vaccine developed from urine to treat and immunize

typhus patients in German concentration camps during forties. That is why hyperthermia should be combined with AUT with or without drugs to achieve this in AIDS.

Effects of Hyperthermia on the Immune System

Hyperthermia causes a rise in white blood cells, including T cell population. This is said to be due to stimulus caused by hyperthermia. At 42° C results in their intense stimulation of lymphocyte production and release (J. Clin. Invest 55:487-499, 1975). Dr. J. R. Downing and his associates have shown that even a mild temperature elevation of 2°C can have dramatic stimulating effect on T cells and interferon gamma and alpha. A modest increase in temperature above 2-3 C is all that is needed to have beneficial effects (The biology of interferon system, Elsevier Science Publications, 1985, P 429). That is why AIDS patients will benefit from moderate to severe hyperthermia treatment using radiant and hot tub methods, instead of going through the deadly, expensive extracorporeal method.

Any investigator interested in treating AIDS should try these methods and may obtain results comparable to severe forms of hyperthermia. The most important part of HIV treatment is to prevent massive destruction of T4 cells and increase T4 cell population to prevent the development of AIDS. Mild to moderate hyperthermia with AUT can achieve this goal.

There is no immediate change in immunoglobulin level. The microbes and affected cells are destroyed or inactivated even by a small amount of antibodies and interferons. Even the small amount of lymphokines stimulate the immune system. But if the urine is fed back during and after hyperthermia, there will be a rise in antibody immunoglobulin levels within ten days. The thermally damaged and inactivated cells are more immunogenic than radiation inactivated cells (Biological and Ultrastructural lesions. Proceedings of international symposium on cancer therapy by hyperthermia and radiation. American College of Radiology press 1976, 3-15). The urine of AIDS patients contain many heat inactivated antigens. Feeding it back stimulates the antibody production against microbes, cofactors, etc. Hyperthermia favorably alters the balance between tumor and host. In the same fashion, it alters favorably towards the host against the AIDS virus.

How Hyperthermia Acts on AIDS Virus, HIV Infected Cells, Opportunistic Infections, Leprosy, Rabies, Tuberculosis, Cancers and other Diseases

1. The lymphocytes and other cells infected with AIDS virus, leprosy and other microorganisms and cancer cells are affected by the heat. It increases cell metabolism many hundred folds. It causes anaerobic cell respiration and anaerobic sugar breakdown (glycolysis). This results in production of acids in the cell. These acids and heat increase lysosomal (a kind of incinerator within the cell) activity. This results in cell death. As the cell dies, its contents are released into circulation and come out in the urine. They are fed back. These tumor cells, AIDS and rabies virus, leprosy and tuberculosis bacteria, etc., are denatured by heat and digestive enzymes, and act as antigens. These antigens are absorbed and stimulate the synthesis of antibodies, which act against diseases and disease causing organisms (Fig.7).
2. Heat suppresses ribonucleic acid (RNA) protein synthesis systems. Without RNA synthesis, the cells cannot survive. AIDS and rabies viruses cannot reproduce without RNA synthesis (because they are RNA viruses). Heat inhibits production of HIV virus by inhibiting reverse transcriptase enzyme like AZT, ddI etc. Heat also inhibits the multiplication of various other bacteria and parasites, including lepra and tuberculosis bacteria.
3. Dr. R. A. Lambert's studies on the hanging drop cultures showed that the normal cells could tolerate temperature up to 6 hours and sarcoma cells for 3 hours at 43°C. The hotter the media, the less time is required for the heat to be effective against tumor or microbes. Heat at 43°C, inactivates chromosomal proteins. At 45°C or more, proteins within the cells begin to coagulate. If the heat is raised up to 45°C, the AIDS virus within cell genes also dies with the cell. In the same fashion, cancer and other incurable diseases are also

eliminated. But at this temperature, even the healthy cells die. Death ensures due to failure of vital organs. That is why it is important to maintain the temperature at 41.8 ° C or below.

4. The cancer cells, the cells infected with AIDS virus, microbes causing opportunistic infections and other diseases like leprosy, rabies and tuberculosis are sensitive to heat. The cell membrane of these disease infected cells is defective. Because it contains part of HIV other microbe material shed when they enter or exit the cell. The heat literally disrupts the defective cell membrane and leaks its contents into circulation. These contents come out in the urine. These denatured contents, when taken orally, are further denatured by the digestive juices and absorbed. They act as antigens, stimulating the immune system against cancers, AIDS, leprosy, tuberculosis, opportunistic infections, etc.

5. All the investigators on hyperthermia have concentrated their research on the effects of elevated temperature on microbes and cancer cells. They have ignored the benefits of heat associated turbulent rapid blood, lymph, and interstitial fluid flow. They also have totally ignored the effects of heat on intercellular spaces, which enhances or facilitates the entrance and exit of substances, antibodies, antigens, humoral factors and immune defence cells from lymphatics and blood vessels. They do not even mention the possible detachment of macromolecules from the surface of vessels and cell walls, due to heat and turbulent fluid flows. In the same fashion, the benefits of exercise are also due to turbulent rapid forceful blood flow, and elevated temperature at the cellular level as described below.

During hyperthermia, the blood and lymph flow becomes turbulent and circulation increases in every organ and around every cell in the body. It can be compared to the rapid waters of the Colorado river which smashes, erodes and moves everything on its way, compared to a quiet Mississippi river. The blood passing through various organs and each cell increases by 3-5 times. In this rapid flow, the cells are churned up. The weak cells and microbes die. Various components attached or deposited in the blood and lymph vessel wall and cells are detached and enter the circulation. These components containing blood enter kidneys and come out as filtrate in the urine. The urine contains large amounts of these liberated substances. This rapid blood flow enhances the output of various substances which otherwise would not have come out including microbes causing opportunistic infections.

The heat and the increased speed of blood enhances the macromolecule of the cells and in between the tissue to get loosened and facilitate their entrance into blood and lymph circulation. It is like steam washing an automobile engine. The urine in these patients is rich in these heat denatured substances. This results in tremendous out pouring of substances which act as antigens and building material. These antigens and other substances taken back orally stimulate the production of different kinds of antibodies which can cure or curtail diseases and help to build vigorous body immune defenses.

6. Hyperthermia (as well as exercise) increases, but severe hyperthermia for long periods depresses the lymphocytes production. These cells enhance the immune system and attack the disease causing organisms. Studies in rats have shown that the natural killer lymphocytes (NK) cells activity increases when the temperature is raised to 40° C. The heat enhances the process of lymphocyte production, maturation and their liberation into circulation. The blood contains healthy, young, disease-free lymphocytes. These lymphocytes breath life into the dead or dying immune system and fight the disease and the offending organisms. That is why it is important to undergo moderate hyperthermia treatment if a person is HIV positive. These people may live healthy without developing AIDS, if combined with AUT. You may eliminate the HIV infection from the body completely. Due to turbulent circulation the leprosy bacillus (killed or denatured) hiding in the nerve sheath gets flushed out into the circulation to be attacked by the immune system.
7. Hyperthermia (and exercise) produces turbulent blood flow in the red bone marrow, liver, thymus gland, spleen, blood

vessels, nervous system, lymph nodes and vessels. Because of the turbulent flow of blood and lymph, the young lymphocytes, trapped in the web of bone marrow, lymph nodes, spleen, liver, thymus gland, and other organs are released. This results in elevated white blood cells during hyperthermia. Thus young healthy lymphocytes free of the infection enter circulation. These lymphocytes enhance the immune system and attack diseases and disease-causing agents including AIDS Virus.

8. During hyperthermia, there is a tremendous increase in demand for oxygen because of enhanced enzyme activity within the cells. This results in an oxygen deficit and produces a state of hypoxia. This further results in increased the production of white blood cells and red blood cells. The whole blood is teaming with new cells ready to fight the diseases.
9. Heat sensitizes disease-afflicted cells and the disease causing organisms to such a level, that even a small amount of antimicrobial or anticancer drugs or radiation, interferons and antibodies can become effective without adversely affecting healthy cells. Heat achieves this by altering the cell membranes of the disease afflicted cells and microbes.
10. Heat has adverse effect on microbes. Their coating is softened and will not latch on to the receptor sites easily to enter the cells and cause diseases, e.g., T4 cells by AIDS virus. The weakened cell membrane of the microbes and the infected cells allows the immune system to recognize these microbes and destroy them. The toxins they produce are inactivated by heat. Heat wrecks the entire machinery of the microbes and the tumor cells. This results in production of less amount of least effective toxins. It also results in reduced multiplication of genetically altered, less toxic, and non-disease producing (less virulent) organisms and cells.
11. Hyperthermia increases blood and lymph circulation and it's force, which detaches some of the components of disease causing microbes and disease afflicted cells. This will make the immune system recognize these disease-afflicted cells and microbes and destroy them.

12. Heat, elevated blood pressure, and rapid turbulent blood flow loosens the connection between the cells of the blood vessels and lymph vessels. It also removes and/or loosens the amorphous material deposits between the cells. This will allow the entry and exit of immune defence cells and humoral factors enter and exit with ease. This will facilitate proper functioning of the immune cells. Immune system to be effective, the cell should be able to move to the site of the disease. Hyperthermia helps this processes. Because of the removal of the intercellular obstruction, antibodies, humoral factors, and immune defence cells can reach the site of the disease easily. They can also move the offending material from the site of insult with ease.
13. Hyperthermia breaks the blood brain barrier which prevents the entrance of many drugs into the brain. Thus it can help in the treatment on many diseases affecting the brain and other parts of the nervous system, such as Alzheimer disease, Parkinson disease, senile dementia, rabies, leprosy, viral fungal and bacterial infections, etc. Hyperthermia will flush out the AIDS virus (and other bacteria) and its components which are bound to the brain cells and glial cells affecting their function and causing brain cell death. I do believe that the rabies can be cured by hyperthermia combined with autoimmune urine therapy, critical care and life support. Please give my facilities an opportunity. I have better than a 50% possibility of curing people with AIDS, rabies, leprosy tuberculosis, etc. Or try what I recommend in this book.
14. Heat, turbulent and rapid blood, and lymph flow detaches and loosens all the cofactors of a disease. Cofactors are many kinds of substances such as proteins, microbes, drugs, chemicals, etc., which make a viruses or microbes and other factors produce diseases. One such cofactor recently identified is a mycoplasma bacteria, which is found in many AIDS patients. HTLV-I and II, HHV-6, hepatitis C viruses, spirocheta, foreign proteins, etc., are also implicated as cofactors. They are all transmitted the same way as the AIDS virus. They are not found in healthy humans. Dr. Luc Montagnier of Pasteur institute found mycoplasma organism in

37 out of 97 patients infected with AIDS virus. Red blood cell infected with mycoplasma can kill white blood cells, thus reducing the immune defense, contributing to AIDS.

AIDS virus is said to produce diseases because of the cofactors. Many of these cofactor are neutralized by heat. Hyperthermia kills the red blood cells infected with mycoplasma and other cofactors. They all come out in the urine. When the are fed back, they produce large amounts of antibodies against them. Combining heat therapy with AUT removes all the cofactors of AIDS and other diseases, resulting in cure or curtailing the disease. Research should be directed at finding an antibiotic which will work against mycoplasma cofactor also. The present antibiotics are not that effective. AUT will produce antibodies which will eliminate mycoplasma infection cofactor.

15. Plasma endorphins, which are similar in function to morphine, go up in blood during hyperthermia, reducing the pain in the body.

An explanation of how hyperthermia and autoimmune urine therapies act in AIDS is described in Chapter 9, 18. Many of the explanations given there also apply to cancers and incurable diseases.

Hyperthermia Like Benefits of Exercise

According to Aerobic Guru Dr. Kenneth Cooper, sedentary lifestyle is defined as anyone who gets less than 20 minutes of aerobic exercise three times a week. Exercise reduces the risk of heart attack and cancers, helps to control the weight problem, high blood pressure and cholesterol and adds years to your life. When it comes to heart attacks, I believe that the lack of exercise is the single most important risk factor compared to other risk factors such as diet, smoking, high blood pressure, overweight, high cholesterol and family history of heart attack.

Exercise physiologist including Dr. Cooper have totally ignored the benefits of hyperthermia like effects of exercise. All of them talk of getting the benefits due to aerobic effects and increased strength of the heart, muscles, lungs and the bones. A stronger heart can pump blood more efficiently for a longer time and is less prone to heart attack. What about other changes that take place during exercise? What about the changes at cellular levels such as:

1. Increased blood flow.
2. Turbulent blood and lymph flow.
3. Dilatation of blood vessels.
4. Increase in spaces between the blood and lymph vessel linings.
5. Transfer material between the tissues and through these spaces.
6. Transfer and transport of substances between the cells and the vessels.
7. Movement of immune system cells and humoral factors.
8. Detachment of macromolecules from the blood vessel wall and cells in the body.
9. Increase in out put of carbon dioxide due to enhanced metabolism.
10. Increased production of lymphocytes and red blood cells.
11. One of the reasons the people who exercise experience fewer heart attacks is that the rapid turbulent heated blood flow cleans the blood vessels of atherosclerotic deposits. That is why I say that exercise is like having a mild to moderate hyperthermia. Due to this reason, the people with AIDS and other incurable diseases should exercise to live longer brought on by above factors. Mild and moderate hyperthermia as prescribed in this chapter can prevent development of atherosclerotic heart and blood vessel diseases. People afflicted with minor angina can get relief without going through expensive angioplasty and open heart coronary artery by pass surgery by mild to moderate hyperthermia. Increased heart rate may cause increase in chest pain. The pain will be reduced gradually with multiple treatments. This procedure may have to be done under physician supervision if there is marked increase in chest pain and irregular heart beats with hyperthermia.
12. Breaking of blood brain barrier resulting in removal many unwanted substances from the brain which gives a good feeling, restful sleep, as well enhances our mental power.

Many other changes exercise brings are similar to the changes seen in hyperthermia as described in this chapter and other chapters (Chapter 9, 14, 18) in this book. All these changes are responsible for reducing the heart attacks and cancers and add years to our life.

The heart may beat irregularity during severe exercise. This is probably due to low magnesium levels in the blood as seen in hyperthermia. It is likely that the athletes who die while playing strenuous games such as basketball, running, football, etc., may be due to low levels of magnesium and phosphates, in addition to the stress resulting in irregular heart beating and sudden death (ventricular fibrillation). The athletes with irregular heart beat should get tested for magnesium levels in the blood.

Broken Blood Brain Barrier by Hyperthermia

It is interesting to note that the blood vessels in the brain do not allow certain substances to enter the nerve cells of the brain. This is called blood brain barrier. During hyperthermia, this barrier is broken and allows many substances that could not enter the brain otherwise. In the same fashion, during exercise, the blood brain barrier is breached to some extent, allowing the substances into the brain otherwise could not have entered. Some of the metabolic products enter the brain, which will not be allowed inside the brain otherwise. The good sleep we get after full day of labor and rigorous exercise may be due to entrance of certain substances which act on the brain and make it rest. That is why after heavy work, exercise, working in the sun and fever, you develop lassitude and get a restful sleep. Other reasons are that phosphate and magnesium levels also go down in blood plasm. This is said to be due to transfer of the ions into the cells. This results in production of lassitude and even irregular heart beat. The breaking of the blood brain barrier has many implications in health and disease. This is one of the reason I believe, hyperthermia can reduce the agony and time spent going through the withdrawal state after stopping the addicting agents such as drugs, alcohol, tobacco, etc.

Forms of Hyperthermia

Three forms of hyperthermia have been developed for treating diseases. Unless specified, hyperthermia means, whole body hyperthermia.

1. **Local:** Heating only the tumor locally.

2. **Regional:** Heating a sector of the body, including the area affected, such as an extremities or intestines etc.

3. **Whole body:** Heating the entire body to treat generalized diseases such as AIDS which affects all organs and wide spread cancers.

Methods of Hyperthermia

Several kinds of energies and methods are used to produce hyperthermia. They are: heated water, electromagnetic energy from radio frequency, microwave, sonic energy from ultrasound, scattered light from infrared light and laser energy from the Nd:YAG laser, radiant heat; heated water, air, and wax; fever producing malarial parasite and bacterial product injection.

1. **Bacterial and Malarial Parasite injection:** Before the turn of the century, bacterial products, and later malarial parasites were injected to produce fever (heat).
2. **Immersing the whole body in hot wax:** hyperthermia induction by giving heated nitrous oxide, carbon dioxide, and oxygen to breathe under general anesthesia and immersing the patient in heated wax (Pettigrew RT et al. Br J Surg 4: 679, 1974).
3. **Wearing a water heated suit or blanket:** Heating the body with automatic temperature controlled water heated suits (Bull JM. et al. Ann Int Med 90:317, 1979).
4. **Immersing in hot water:** The whole body is immersed in hot water to achieve the desired temperature (Sladen A, et al. Clin. Res. 31, 2601 A, 1981)

5. **Extracorporeal heating (Fig.1):** Blood is removed from the femoral artery in the groin, heated by a water heated exchange coil. The heated blood is put back into the body through the femoral vein. The body is enclosed in a nonconducting blanket and the procedure is done under general anesthesia (Parks LC et al. J Thorac. Cardiovasc. Surg 78:883, 1979).
6. **Hot air + water mattress or diathermy:** Externally applied Siemens box or modified Siemens box (Pomp H. Cancer therapy by hyperthermia and radiation, Urban and Schwarzenberg, 1978, p326).
7. **Radiant heat using specially designed chamber to produce radiant heat (Fig.2):** This procedure is safer, non-invasive and can be done under sedation (Robins HI et al. J clinc Oncol 2: 1050, 1984).
8. **Local hyperthermia:** Heating locally for cancers is becoming common. Many technical advances are made in equipment and the heating source. Microwave, radio frequency, ultrasound, laser and thermometry equipment are used to produce heat locally.

Method 1, 2, 3, and 5 are rarely used. Extracorporeal heating (Method 5) is expensive, labor intensive, and associated with life-threatening complications, such as anesthesia mishaps, bleeding, infection, air embolus, technical failure, etc. It requires a team of vascular surgeons, cardiopulmonary bypass technicians (perfusionist) and well-trained anesthesiologists. I believe that this method of hyperthermia should be discouraged.

Heating the whole body by radiant heat (method 7) should be tried. This method is safer, less expensive, less invasive, does not need any general anesthesia, can be done under sedation, decreased complications, improved patient comfort, cost effective, patient remains responsive and does not need a team of highly trained medical personnel. If the disease is localized, local or regional hyperthermia should be used instead of whole body hyperthermia.

DO IT YOURSELF HOME HYPERTHERMIA

Sauna, Steam Room and Hot Water Hyperthermia: A Method to Increase the Body Temperature without going to a Physician

Hyperthermia is still experimental and is becoming an adjunct therapy rather than a primary method of cure. I do believe that when it is practiced along with autoimmune urine therapy (AUT), drugs and other modern medical therapies, it can cure or curtail diseases, prolong life, ease pain and suffering. It is likely that in AIDS patients we may not have to bring the temperature up to 41. 8° C. All they need is exposure to heat in a sauna about 1-3° C higher than the normal body temperature for 2-3 times a week, lasting 1-2 hours at a time. There are only limited number of places where hyperthermia is induced for advanced cancers. It is going to take years to establish it as a therapy for various diseases, including AIDS.

A person who has a deadly disease needs help now, not tomorrow. I do recommend people who want to involve in their own therapy should try my hot water immersion, steam room or dry sauna method. As I stated before, to stimulate the lymphocytes and immune system, one has to undergo heat therapy for 2-3 hours above 2-3° C normal body temperature. Heating the body using extracorporeal method is not needed. Mild to moderate hyperthermia can be induced by entering into dry sauna, steam room or hot water immersion in hot tub or heated jacuzzi with high temperature settings. There are a number of preparation to be done before starting this therapy.

The following guidelines will help you to start your own hyperthermia program at home. This can help those suffering from AIDS, HIV positive, and other incurable diseases.

How Much Time Should a Person Stay in the Dry Sauna?

I classify hyperthermia into 3 groups according to the body temperature.

1. **Mild hyperthermia:** Body temperature up to 38. 5°C. Mild hyperthermia of short duration may stimulate both the microbes and cancer cells. This effect is off set by above described beneficial effects. Using only mild hyperthermia is not sufficient. It should be combined with the AUT and drugs.

2. **Moderate hyperthermia:** Body temperature up to 40°C. This method should be tried before resorting to severe hyperthermia in AIDS and for other acute and chronic diseases.
3. **Severe hyperthermia:** Body temperature up to 41. 8°C. This method should be tried if there is no improvement by above methods combined with AUT.

The following table gives some guidelines about the time spent in hot water, steam room or sauna. It should be adjusted according to the condition of the patient and the disease.

Week	Hours (hr) in sauna or hot water after reaching the set temp.	How many times a week
First week	½-1 hr	2
Second week	1½ hr	2
Third week	2-2½ hr	1
fourth week	2½ hr	once every two weeks
Sixth week	3 hr	once every fourth week
Tenth week	3-4 hr	once every sixth week

Weekly practice of getting into the sauna at an enjoyable temperature should continue for many months. After the above regimen is completed, try to stay in the sauna, steam roon or hot water for 2-4 hours with desired temperature settings every three months once. Once you achieve the body temperature of 108°F, stay in the sauna or hot water for the desired amount of time. Do not go above this body temperature. The sauna temperature sets up to 198 °F. This has to be cut down so that the body temperature does not go beyond 108° F.

Thermal Runaway

It is important to remember that the heat increases the body metabolism. The increased metabolism produces heat within the body. This will result in what we call the "thermal runaway" phenomenon, if it is not properly controlled by lowering the sauna, steam roon or hot water temperature setting. Such a runaway temperature can be deadly. It usually takes up to 90 minutes to reach the desired temperature and about 30 to 50 minutes to bring it down. The skin has an area of 1.7 square meters, whereas the lungs has 20 times the area of skin. Thus inhaling the heated air and skin coming in contact with the radiant heat or hot water can raise the core body temperature fast. As the body temperature reaches up to 41. 8°C, bring the head through the modified sauna door and reduce the sauna or hot water temperature to no more than 44. 5°C (112°F).

Modification of Sauna or Steam Room Door

At times it may be difficult to control the temperature of the body inside the sauna chamber. This may result in an increase in the body temperature to dangerous levels. To prevent any such mishaps, the door of the sauna need to be modified. A tight hole, the size that will allow the head to project out of the door easily, should be cut. The hole should be provided with tight shutters to be used in the initial phase of hyperthermia to keep the door shut. A soft collar is provided in the cut door shutters to seal around the patient's neck. The soft collar also permits the passage of the intravenous fluid lines, and monitoring cables into the chamber (Fig.2).

The patient undergoing hyperthermia therapy lays on a movable bench or stretcher. The body is wrapped in a plastic sheet and covered with thick blankets. This will prevent the body from loosing fluids and temperature from the skin by evaporation. The head is pulled out through the door outside the sauna or steam room chamber. By this method, the vital signs and the temperature can be monitored. If the temperature climbs up beyond 41. 8°C, move one of the extremities through the hole in the door till the temperature drops. Once the temperature drops to the desired level, put the extremity back inside the chamber. If the body temperature falls below the level, make the patient breath hot air from the sauna or electric heater forced hot air. This is one of the safest method of achieving the desired temperature.

If the person has their head projecting out of the sauna door, there is a possibility of loosing heat due to rapid breathing of cold air. To prevent it, attach a 1-2 inch diameter rubber or plastic breathing tube with a tight fitting mask around the face. These plastic tubing and the face mask can be obtained from medical equipment supply stores everywhere. Connect the distal end inside the sauna chamber and the proximal end around the face mask. Snorkeling equipment can be adopted to breath hot air from the sauna or any heated air source. By this method, the patient will breath hot air and will not loose temperature. Whenever the temperature raises more than the set level, breathe room air till the desired temperature is reached. Many of the AIDS patients are well educated and very smart. They can use their ingenuity to solve any problem that may arise during home hyperthermia.

Preparation for Home Hyperthermia

1. Equipment needed:
   a. Carry two thermometers. One to take oral temperature and the other to take rectal temperature. The temperature probes can be attached to the body and carried outside the sauna chamber to measure the temperature. Because of the intense heat within the sauna chamber, the thermometers may not record the correct temperature. The temperature probes may have to be passed through the peep whole as they are needed. Monitor the hot water temperature by an ordinary thermometer from hardware store.
   b. Electric heating plate to keep the drinking fluids hot. Do not use natural gas to heat.

c. Plenty of plain water, and gatorade. Do not use any alcoholic drinks or addictive drugs in the sauna chamber. Do not smoke.
d. Carry clean plastic and linens sheets, and towels.
e. Keep 2-3 clean drinking glasses to collect urine and drink, and to be used for drinking water.
f. Have intercom system or phone (cordless if available) where you can communicate with people outside and inform them of your condition.
g. Have a nonabsorbent pillow or towel as pillow.
h. The wooden movable bench covered with soft padding inside the sauna should be able to support you sitting and should be able let you lay down comfortably.

2. Always have one or two people to watch you. Have vehicle available for emergency transportation. Install surveillance camera with video cassette recording to document the procedure for future analysis.
3. One member of the team watching you should be trained in cardiopulmonary resuscitation (CPR).
4. Make sure that the observers record all the data you send out. It is hard to write in the sauna or hot tub because of profuse sweating. You can use a tape to record the changes in temperature and condition.
5. Carry a stopwatch. Install a big wall clock outside the sauna chamber which you can see through the door. Make sure the sauna is well lighted and has a two-way visible glass door.
6. Have radio and other audio visual equipment of your choice. Rent a movie of your choice so that you can pass time within the sauna or hot water with ease.
7. Have a cylinder of oxygen, an Ambu bag to ventilate, oral airway, automatic BP measuring device (Dinamap), pulse oximeter which measures O_2 saturation and expiratory carbon dioxide output monitoring device (capnograph) and electrocardiogram (EKG) with a tape to record the heart beats. This equipment is a must for severe hyperthermia and difficult to use during hot water tub hyperthermia. They may not be

needed for mild to moderate hyperthermia and severe hyperthermia of short duration.

8. If a person wants to a stay long time under high temperature settings in the sauna, sedatives, tranquilizers, barbiturates, valium, etc., need to administered under physician supervision to prevent anxiety, and agitation created by hyperthermia. Do not take aspirin. It can aggravate the bleeding condition.

CAUTION: Electronic equipment may malfunction due to intense heat in sauna and hot water tubs. In such cases, the monitors should be used outside. Keep oxygen tank outside the sauna chamber.

The Day before Sauna, Steam Room or Hot Water Hyperthermia

1. Fast at least one to two days before and practice Total Autoimmune urine therapy (TAUT).
2. Drink only water and all the urine passed.
3. Do not take any medications except specific and antimicrobial or anticancer drugs. Sedatives may be needed if you are undergoing severe hyperthermia.
4. Take a mild shower, wash your hair and brush your teeth with urine before going to bed.
5. Do not eat any breakfast.
6. Rest well and get a good night sleep.
7. Go through the routine with your friends and loved ones. Make sure they are immediately available in seconds.

The Day of Hyperthermia Exposure

1. Take a mild shower.
2. Set the temperature in the sauna to 99° C (196°F) and hot water temperature at 112°F.
3. Take all your equipment and supplies inside sauna.
4. Enter the sauna or hot water tubs.
5. Record the temperature every 15 minutes orally and/or rectally. Once the desired temperature is achieved (takes about 50-90 minutes), lower the sauna or hot water temperature setting to your body temperature level plus or minus 3°F.

6. Keep people moving in and out of the sauna or bath room to the minimum to maintain the steady temperature in the chamber.
7. Stay in the chamber or hot tubs according to your need. See the table above and set your guide lines. Stay about 2-4 hours total or about 2-4 hours once the body reaches 108° F temperature to achieve severe hyperthermia.
8. Drink plenty of water and all the urine. Do not drink cold water. Drink water heated to 100 to 102°F on the heating plate. Start intravenous fluids with the help of paramedic or nurse or physician. Administer 5% warm glucose in 0. 45% normal saline solution at the rate of 500 to 750 ml per hour if you are undergoing severe hyperthermia.
9. Try to breath slowly. As the body heat raises, the respiratory rate goes up. This may result in what we call respiratory alkalosis. This can cause blood acid - base (pH) derangement, electrolyte abnormality, neuromuscular irritability manifesting as tetany and carpopedal spasm. Administer oxygen 2-6 liters per minute using nasal canula in cases of sever hyperthermia and patients with lung diseases.
10. Monitor the temperature every 15 minute once, both rectally and orally. Blood pressure and temperature monitoring is all that is needed for mild to moderate hyperthermia.
11. For severe hyperthermia, monitor BP, carbon dioxide output in expired air (end tidal CO2), oxygen saturation (SpO2), and EKG continuously. Make sure your friends know how to use and interpret these electronic monitors. You may have to get the help of a nurse or nurse anesthetist or a physician to read these monitors. It may be difficult to use many of these monitoring devices in hot water tub hyperthermia. Normal O_2 saturation is 99-100%. life can be sustained at 70-75% saturation. ETCO2 reading should be about 28-35 mm Hg. You are breathing too fast if it falls below 24 mm Hg and breathing too slow if it is above 45 mm Hg. Continuously monitor EKG in all severe hyperthermia. If any heart irregularity develops, the procedures need to be discontinued and seek a physicians or emergency room help immediately.

The following table gives the temperature in centigrade and Fahrenheit:

Temperature Conversion Table

Fahrenheit	Centigrade	Fahrenheit	Centigrade
98.6	37.0	104.0	40.0
99.0	37.2	105.0	40.5
100.0	37.7	106.0	41.1
101.0	38.3	107.0	41.7
102.0	38.0	108.0	42.2
103.0	39.4	109.0/112.1	42.8/44.5
149.0/156.0	78.0/80.0	196.0	99.0

The following formula allows you to convert the temperature from C to F and vice versa: C= (F-32)x 5/9. F= (Cx9/5) + 32.

12. Once you achieve the desired temperature, maintain it for 2-4 hours or what ever your goal is set. Cut down temperature setting of the heating system gradually. Wait till body temperature drops to 99 to 100° F before you come out of the sauna or hot water. Do not drink cold drinks as you come out of sauna or hot water. Continue to drink urine and warm water.
13. Continue urine therapy with total fasting. If not, follow the principals of prophylactic AUT as described in Chapter 8, 9, 10. 11, 18, 19.
14. Rest completely. After hours of sauna, you may feel lassitude for hours and feel better the next day.
15. Follow guidelines given in the following chapters.

The sauna and hot water hyperthermia can eliminate the skin manifestations of AIDS including kaposi. If they are not developed, it will probably prevent their development. If the tests are done on the immune system after 4-10 days, there will be improvements in T_4 cells count. In severe hyperthermia, the lymphocyte count may drop temporarily. Blood levels of AIDS Virus core antigen will drop. The level of antibodies will increase. Practicing this therapy if a person is HIV positive may prevent the development of full blown AIDS. Sauna and hot water hyperthermia can be adopted to treat disease such as leprosy, tuberculosis, rabies, cancers, etc.

Can Hot Water (Tub or Jacuzzi) be Used for Hyperthermia induction?

Hot water has been used to induce local and whole body hyperthermia. Cancers of the male genital organ has been treated by immersing the organ only in hot water by Dr. O. Goetze of Germany in 1932. It is difficult lie down and rest in water for hours. It is difficult to attach the monitoring devices. Get into the hot water with 105°F temperature and then set the inlet water temperature to 112 ° F, about 3-4 degrees higher than what you want to achieve. I have stayed in the bathtub containing hot water at temperature of 112°F up to an hour. Maintain the hot water temperature by slow running, very hot water inlet from the hot water tank. If the immersing water temperature reaches more than 112°F, skin burns can develop. To raise the body temperature rapidly, keep the air surrounding the hot tub that you breath hot by running an electric heater in the bath room.

If a person is suffering from Kaposi sarcoma or the leprosy lesions of the extremities, or trunk, hyperthermia of the skin and subcutaneous tissue can be induced by immersing the body in set hot water set at 112°F. This form of therapy will help to clear the Kaposi's sarcoma of the skin. Get a thermometer from the hardware store and pour a tub full of water, measure and attain the correct temperature, and then immerse your body till desired time. Keep the temperature of the tub water by constantly adding the hot water from your hot water heater. Set the skin temperature no more than 112°F to prevent skin burns.

The entire blood from the body runs through the skin every five minutes during hyperthermia. Thus the AIDS virus and other bacteria in contact with the skin is affected by the skin hyperthermia. The immune system is also gets stimulated. This therapy, you can start it without delay and without a physician advise. There is a good possibility, that the Kaposi's of the skin and leprosy lesions will melt away with this simple therapy. This therapy has to be repeated 2-3 times a week. Follow the skin hyperthermia with external application of urine as described in Chapter 7, 8 and 14.

Regional Hyperthermia

Cancers, or any kind of tumors, skin conditions due to allergy or infection, eczema, leprosy lesions, actinomycosis lesions, bone cancers can be treated with regional hyperthermia. It may not be necessary to subject an individual for total body hyperthermia unless the lesion is spread to other organs. Immerse the limb in hot water or heating jackets. Apply a tourniquet. Squeeze all the blood out of the extremity by elastoplast. Set the tourniquet setting at 25 mm Hg higher than the blood pressure. A medical tourniquet can be obtained from the medical supply house. Learn how to use the tourniquet with the help of surgical nurse or physician. Turn on the tourniquet. Immerse the limb in the hot water set at 105°F, and them gradually add hot water to achieve 112°F. Maintain that temperature by adding the hot water set at that temperature. Achieve the desired level of hyperthermia and maintain the desired amount of time.

If you want to maintain 4-8 hours, the tourniquet has to be let down for 5 minutes and reapplied every 90 minutes. The nerves supplying the area of hyperthermia may need to be blocked by an anesthesiologist if severe hyperthermia is needed for many hours. This blunts the heat sensation. For upper extremity blocking of the brachial plexus, for lower limb blocking of the four nerves (sciatic, femoral, obturator, and lateral cutaneous nerve of the thigh or epidural or low spinal block) will help to sustain the temperature at higher levels with less discomfort. Perineal and genital lesions can be treated by using this method. I wonder sometime that we can treat gas gangrenes, sympathetic dystrophy and other chronic infection using this method. Experiment yourself by immersing one limb in hot water and not the other. See the benefits of it. Kaposis of the leg or the arm can be easily used for this experiment. **I feel that**

that the so called cellulite-ugly skin fat bumps can be eliminated by using tourniquet and hyperthermia method. I am going to experiment on this in near future.

Hyperthermia for Cancer of the Esophagus, Breast, Peritoneal cavity, Rectum, Bladder, -----, ------, ------ ----, ---- -- --- ----- ----, Prostatic hypertrophy, and Other Lesions

There are millions of people suffering from ---------------------------These blank line represents a processes which was described in the original manuscript for which we are applying for a patent which may be able to cure or curtail these conditions in millions of patients-----The details were removed from the galley proofs to prevent other people from coping this procedure.----------------Next edition will contain these details.--------------------etc.

Thousands of people die from food pipe (esophagus) cancer. At present I am designing a heated balloon and to pass it all the way down to the esophagus to the site of lesion and heat the area locally from 108 to 112 to 114 °F. for many hours. During heating, I plan to instill anticancer drugs around the heating element. This will enhance the uptake of these drugs by cancer cells and which act against them and kill them. Further after the local hyperthermia, I am going to inflate a special balloon below the cancer site and fill the rest of the esophagus with anticancer agents and/or morning urine for many hours many times a day. The urine will act locally and systemically. This treatment may have to be repeated many times. This treatment has a better chance of curing or curtailing this cancer. The surgery for cancer of the esophagus results in untold number of complications, pain, miserable life, repeated hospitalization, thousands of dollars in expense and rapid death. Local anesthetics may have to be applied to ease the pain during hyperthermia.

For cancer of the breast, I plan to heat the breast with a special heating pad at 42-44 degree C. Monitor the breast temperature with a probe inserted into the breast mass. Nerve supply to the breast can be blocked by regional anesthesia to ease the pain.

This method can be adopted to prostatic hypertrophy and cancers, rectal cancers, bladder cancers, carcinomatosis of the peritoneal cavity, pancreatic cancers etc.

Fill the peritoneal cavity, rectum, bladder or any other cacity or hollow organ with sterile hot water and maintain it at that temperature with constant water bath. Anticancer agents can be added to the water bath. Repeated applications of this method with AUT will keep the cancer in check, reduce the tumor mass, and may even cure. The treatment has to be repeated many tiems.

The patients and physicians interested in this therapy and starting a research project, please contact me.

Selection of Patients For Hyperthermia: Guidelines

1. Patient should be between 18 to 65 and has exhausted all other modalities of treatment are eligible. For HIV positive and AIDS patient, rabies, leprosy, and tuberculosis, this form of treatment can be started at any age. Start this therapy from the beginning instead of waiting for it to develop into full blown disease with many complications. Children need to be monitored very carefully and time spent in the sauna or hot tubs may have to be tailored.
2. Patient should be psychologically fit. This does not apply to the AIDS patients, because the disease affects the brain at an early stage.
3. Must have projected life span of greater than one month.
4. Must have stable heart and blood vessels (cardiovascular system) because heat creates stress on the heart.
5. Patients with cancer in the brain are not acceptable for severe hyperthermia.

Exceptions for the above criteria can be made depending on the disease and condition of the patient.

Changes in the Body Due to Whole Body Hyperthermia

All these changes takes during severe hyperthermia. These changes are less pronounced during mild and moderate hyperthermia. Many of these changes are also observed during exercise.

1. Hemoglobin: increases in blood due to thermal destruction of old red blood cells (0. 5 to 0. 800/100 cc).

2. Young red blood cells increase (reticulocytosis) between treatments: This indicates bone marrow stimulation by hyperthermia and hypoxia. The platelet count goes down if general anesthesia is given. There are hardly any changes under sedation. That is why it is dangerous to use extracorporeal method to heat under anesthesia. It can cause bleeding disorders.
3. Post and intra treatment rise in bilirubin: indicate liver damage or hemolysis (0. 47 to 0. 62 mg/100 cc)
4. Fluid loss: 550 cc's (20 ounces or about 2½ glasses) of fluid loss per hour in 70 Kg. (160 lb) person of which 90% is lost in the sweat. Calculate the loss and replace it with drinking water. Continue to drink urine. It will eliminate any electrolyte imbalance and at the same time supply nutritive materials and large amount of antigens. For moderate to severe hyperthermia, start an intravenous line and administer 750 ml of 5% dextrose in 0.5% normal saline per hour. Alternate with 5% dextrose with 0. 5% saline with 7.5 mEq/Liter of potassium chloride. KCl addition is reduced or not added if urine therapy is practiced along with the hyperthermia. You need a physicians help to obtain and administer KCl.
5. Increase in white blood cells (leukocytosis) during treatment: as a response to heat and other previously explained factors.
6. Rise in blood pressure. Elevated central venous pressure (CVP) as indicated by prominent bulging neck veins. There is systolic pressure rise of 20-50 mm Hg with little or no change in diastolic pressure. CVP. is elevated by 5-10 cm. H_2O. Heart pumps more blood. In one of our cancer patients the cardiac output went up more than 18 liters per minute. Under normal conditions the heart pumps about 5 liters of blood per minute. That is about 70 cc or 2 ounces per heart beat. (The BP and CVP elevation is due to diminution of impulses from carotid sinus and aortic arch. This leads to increase in sympathetic vasomotor control. This increases the precapillary resistance, resulting in elevated BP, increase venous tone and increased heart rate.)

7. Rise in heart rate: Pulse rate can go up to 180/minute. In the anesthetized patients the elevation is only 60% of the conscious patient. It goes up to 8 to 18 beats per centigrade degree elevation in esophageal temperature.
8. Serum potassium: Rises by 0.5 mEq/L by first 90 minutes of treatment.
9. Serum sodium: Drop by 4.0 mEq/L initially but no change the next 24 hours.
10. Serum chloride usually does not change.
11. Enzymes: No change in LDH, aspartate, alanine aminotransferase. CPK enzyme levels went up after 24 hours of hyperthermia. Alkaline phosphate, SGOT, SGPT, may go up in some cases.
12. Respiration: (↑ =increased, ↓ =decreased).
    ↑ minute volume
    ↑ respiration per minute increases from 11 to 40 at 41. 8°F.
    ↑ O_2 consumption
    ↑ CO_2 excretion
    ↓ CO_2 tension due to hyperventilation. (This is due to heat affecting the carotid body, spinal cord, tongue, and anterior hypothalamus. Atelectasis [collapse of lung alveoli], pulmonary edema and Cheyne-Stokes respiration [irregular breathing] are also observed).
13. Metabolism of tissues: There is increased metabolism at all levels resulting in augmentation of O_2 and glucose consumption, increased CO_2 and heat production at cellular level. Thus the body starts generating its own heat internally. That is why it is important to reduce the temperature of the heating media once the desired temperature is reached.
14. Blood vessel dilatation: Due to heat stimulation of skin sensory responses and liberated local metabolic products act as blood vessels dilator, act on the brain, create poor venous return due to capillary dilatation and venous engorgement.
15. Renal: Decreases the urine output (due to elevated intra renal resistance). If urine therapy is followed, there is normal or increased urine output. Elevated levels of Ca, PO4, and Mg in urine and stools may be due to alkalosis induced by

hyperventilation. No change in serum BUN and creatinine were noted.

16. Brain electrical activity (EEG=electroencephalography): Slow waves with reduced voltage and burst suppression. They also may slow down.
17. Electromyograph (EMG) and nerve conduction studies: Showed slowed conduction (may indicate scattered myelin defect), which returns to normal after a few weeks.
18. Electrocardiogram (EKG): 15% incidence of heart irregularities (arrhythmias) develop under N_2O, O_2 and relaxant anesthesia. When inspiration (FIO_2) of less than 50% oxygen is used, T-wave changes were seen indicating myocardial ischemia. Hyperthermia combined with doxorubicin (Adrimycin, an anticancer agent) results in heart irregularity (PVC's) and drop in BP.
19. There is a decrease in serum phosphate and magnesium. Serum phosphate levels dropped from 3.5 mg/L to as low as 0.6 mg/L and magnesium from 1.7 mEq/L to 1.3 mEq/L. They all returned to normal range by 24 hours. These changes are minimal with AUT.
20. There is a report of exacerbation of multiple sclerosis symptoms (J Nerol Nerosurg Psychatry 22:113-116, 1959). The patients exposed to hyperthermia developed polyneuropathy symptoms within 24 hours after therapy. It is probably caused by neurotoxin and metabolic changes. That is why the patients with multiple sclerosis should try mild to moderate hyperthermia along with AUT instead of severe hyperthermia.

Complications of Whole Body Hyperthermia

Many of these complications occur in sick patients under long periods of severe hyperthermia at 108°F or more. The complications are less likely to happen in young, healthy patients with mild to moderate hyperthermia therapy.

1. Death due to ventricular fibrillation due to rise of temperature to 43°C or more. Low magnesium and phosphate levels can cause heart irregularities as well as nervous system symptoms.
2. Death due to fibrosing alveolitis.

3. Herpes simplex flare up. If urine therapy is followed, they will subside or may not occur. Even if they occur, they will be mild.
4. Sore throat and hoarseness due to endotracheal tube placement under general anesthesia. This will not happen under sedation.
5. Protect pressure areas, including heels, to prevent any pressure sores. Otherwise skin burns are very common.
6. Lassitude (up to 24 hours).
7. Nausea and vomiting.
8. Superficial burns under EKG electrodes.
9. Temperature above 42°C for long period can causes irreversible cell damage.
10. Jaundice due to liver failure.
11. Loss of memory (amnesia).
12. Peripheral neuropathy, foot drop. This is due to low phosphate and magnesium in the blood.
13. Diarrhea. It will not occur if the person fasted for two to three days with AUT.
14. Air trapped between the lungs and rib cage (pneumothorax), lung swelling (pulmonary edema).
15. Increased heart rate (tachycardia) and heart irregularities due to low magnesium levels and high adrenaline out put.
16. Severe bleeding all over the body (low grade disseminated intravascular clotting with elevated fibrinogen split products).
17. Muscle tissue breakdown (rhabdomyolysis with elevated CPK of 40, 000 I. U).
18. Patients undergoing repeated heat exposures will not experience cumulative toxicity.

The following guidelines were followed in our hospital hyperthermia program:

Tests Done Before Subjecting to Hyperthermia

The following tests are usually done a day before hyperthermia and anesthesia. Many of the tests can be ruled out on the basis of physical examination by the physician. Mild to moderate hyperthermia may not need most of these tests and monitoring discussed. **Temperature recording is a must in all the cases.**

1. 12 Lead EKG.
2. Creatine phosphokinase (CPK) isoenzyme before and 24 hours after hyperthermia.
3. Echocardiogram: to know the size of heart chambers and to rule out any fluid in the heart sac (pericardial effusion).
4. Chest x-ray: before and after hyperthermia.
5. SMA 18 blood analysis (Blood chemistry and electrolytes).
6. Electrolytes such as potassium, calcium, phosphates, magnesium, zinc, chloride.
7. Brain CAT scan to rule out any tumors. Death can ensue under hyperthermia due to necrosis and edema of the brain caused by breaking of the blood brain barrier.
8. Patient should be free of any limiting cardiovascular diseases. No mitral valve prolapse to be included because they can't sustain the stress of elevated cardiac output. They need to be closely monitored if severe hyperthermia is used. They can probably tolerate mild to moderate hyperthermia.
9. Bleeding time, PTT, PT, platelet count (never less than 75000/mm3), CPK, LDH, alkaline phosphatase, Ca, Mg, urea nitrogen, creatinine.
10. Hemoglobin: at least 10 g.
11. Electromyogram and nerve conduction studies.
12. Abdominal distension and ascites are to be ruled out because of danger of vomiting and aspiration.
13. Lung function tests: preoperative blood gases, FEV1 to be 60% or greater, vital capacity to be at least 50% of the predicted.
14. Kidney function assessed by creatine clearance test.
15. Patient does not eat after midnight the day before procedure to prevent any aspiration of the stomach contents during and after the procedure.

Patient Monitoring during Hyperthermia

You need the help of a nurse, physician assistant or physician to monitor some of the below monitors. These monitors are not needed for all cases. Some of the hyperthermia methods need only simple monitoring of temperature, blood pressure, urine output, which can be monitored easily. Of all the methods of hyperthermia, the extracorporeal method needs the most monitoring because this method is complicated and dangerous.

1. Temperature: esophageal, rectal, skin (2 places), tympanic if possible.
2. EKG: back pad and five lead.
3. Respiratory rate.
4. Tidal and minute volume: by spirometer and mask.
5. End expiratory CO_2 ($ETCO_2$).
6. Swan Ganz catheter with thermodilution port to monitor pulmonary artery pressure, temperature, and cardiac output.
7. Radial arterial blood pressure needed for extracorporeal method only or in critically ill patients.
8. Arterial, mixed venous (SVO2, pulmonary artery) and forearm venous O2 and CO2 gas measurement.
9. Urine output (hourly) by using Foley catheter.
10. Electroencephalogram (EEG) - for cerebral function.
11. Blood pressure cuff to arm with forearm venous line to evaluate the blood gases of venous blood.
12. Use warming blankets to maintain the elevated temperature and minimize the heat loss.

Many of these tests and monitoring devices are not needed in healthy patients done under sedation without using extracorporeal circulation.

Temperature Monitoring during Hyperthermia

For simple and moderate hyperthermia, monitor only oral, esophageal or rectal and skin temperatures.

1. Optimal temperature for severe hyperthermia is 41. 8° C.
2. Temperature greater than 42 C. can cause irreversible cell damage or death.
3. To raise temperature from 37° C to 41° C in a 70 Kg man requires 280, 000 calories of heat.
4. Body skin has 1. 5 square meters body surface area, whereas lungs have 20 times (30 square meters) the surface area. This

can result in great loss of temperature by breathing. That is why the anesthetic gases or breathing air are heated to prevent heat loss.

5. Skin temperature should not go above 44° C.
6. Esophageal temperature should never exceed 41. 8° C and rectal 42° C.
7. Esophageal probe is placed at lower fourth of esophagus, below the level of great vessels.
8. Rectal probe passed between 10 to 20 cm. into rectum.
9. Tympanic temperature (through the external ear, measured by a special probe) if needed measures brain temperature indirectly.
10. Pulmonary artery temperature by Swan Ganz catheter measures the temperature of the blood inside the heart.

Anesthetic Techniques (A Guide for Physicians)

Total body severe hypothermia (41.8° C) can be done under general anesthesia or sedation. The following are some of the methods used at various centers. It is important to remember that the general anesthesia inhibits the immune system temporarily. Any hyperthermia procedure advocating general anesthesia should be avoided.

1. Lee, et al (Anesthesiology, 52: 418-428, 1980).

   Plan A: Thiopental 7± 3 mg/Kg/Hour. Fentanyl 3± 1 ug/Kg/Hour. Total dose of thiopental 3 grams and fentanyl (a potent narcotic) 800 ug. Spontaneous ventilatory pattern activity maintained. **Plan B:** Innovar 0. 2 ml/Kg/Hour. Helped to maintain normal carbon dioxide and oxygen level. It causes hypotension during hyperthermia induction due to the droperidol component of innovar. Elevation of body temperature augments the alpha blocking effect of droperidol. The patient was not intubated.

   Plan C: Sodium pentothal 5 mg/Kg. initially,25 - 100ug/Kg/Min, subsequently by drip. Total dose 2 grams. No intubation.

2. Pettigrew WRT, et al (Br. Med J 4: 679-682, 1974). Premedicate with Thorazine. I. V. Barbiturates, Paralyzed by curare and given heated nitrous oxide and oxygen
3. Bull JM, et al (Ann Intern Med 90: 317-323, 1979). Ketamine 25 ug/Kg/Min or Sodium Pentothal 100 ug/Kg/Min drip combined with Fentanyl 0.05 ug/Kg/Min drip. No intubation, spontaneous breathing. Thermally induced hyperventilation, if not controlled results in respiratory alkalosis, tetany, neuromuscular irritability. Ketamine may cause more heat loss due to stimulation of breathing (ventilation).
4. Robins HI, et al (Int. J. Radiation Oncology Biol, Phys. 18: 909-920, 1990). They have induce hyperthermia under sedation using radiant heat method without using extremely complicated dangerous extracorporeal method. They gave intravenous pentothal (4mg/minute), lidocaine (4 mg/minute). They also gave IV droperidol (2-5mg), diazepam (valium 2-5mg), and fentanyl (25-50μg) as needed. Patients go to their room and do not need intensive care. Foley catheter is used to monitor urine output.

Halothane or other halogenated anesthetic agents should not be used to prevent any heart irregularities (arrhythmias) and liver damage. Patient may develop Cheyne-Stokes respiration. Lee, et al treated it with increasing barbiturate drip. Barbiturates also have a protective effect on the brain.

Anesthetic method Used in Georgia Baptist Medical Center, Atlanta, by Dr. T. R. Shantha M.D,Ph.D, in 1981 Cancer Hyperthermia Studies

1. Narcotic + Barbiturate combination.
2. Heated N_2O + O_2 were used.
3. Repeated doses of non depolarizing muscle relaxants are needed to be administered at short intervals. We used curare to relax the ventilatory muscles and control the respiration. It is metabolized quickly due to hyperthermia. May require up to 150 mg of curare in two hours.

4. Patients were intubated. Controlled respiration. Inspiratory gases humidified and heated.
5. Premedicated with Innovar. No Atropine was given. We gave large amounts of potassium phosphate to maintain proper serum phosphates. If Total AUT is followed this my not be needed. They may need magnesium to prevent heart irregularities.

It is becoming clear that the patients should not be given general anesthesia for hyperthermia because it depresses the immune system and creates bleeding problems. Hyperthermia that uses radiant heat without any anesthesia should be used instead of the extracorporeal method.

Precautions during Hyperthermia Procedure

1. Cover the eyes.
2. Cover hair with swim cap.
3. Cover ears with cotton wool.
4. All pressure points (occiput, sacrum, ischium, elbows, head, scapula, etc.) should be well protected by padding.
5. Soda lime carbon dioxide absorber must be functional and checked constantly to prevent CO_2 accumulation if general anesthesia is used.

Maintenance of Fluids Given Intravenously during Severe Hyperthermia

Mild to moderate hyperthermia of short duration may not need intravenous fluid administration. Long periods of moderate and severe hyperthermia needs fluid administration through a vein according the following guidelines. If AUT is practiced, the urine can be fed through the small stomach feeding tube. In such cases reduce the dose of fluids taking into account the amount of urine administered.

1. 500 to 750 ml/hour Dextrose in water. Alternate with 0.45 saline with 10 to 20 mEq/L of KCl (Bull, et al). If AUT is practiced, KCl may not be needed.
2. 0.45 Physiologic saline with 5% dextrose at the rate of 10-15 cc/Kg/Hour (Lee, et al).

3. Maintenance of osmolarity at slightly higher level helps to prevent the fluid (accumulation) retention in lungs. This is done by giving 1.8% saline.
4. There is elevated metabolism, so glucose solutions need to be given.
5. Urine output below 75 cc/hour should be treated with lasix (furosemide). When urine is used to be fed back, this is not needed. AUT stimulates the urine output.

I hope this book will stimulate interest in hyperthermia as a adjunct method of treatment for other diseases besides cancer such as: AIDS, leprosy, tuberculosis, rabies, autoimmune diseases, skin diseases, atherosclerotic blood vessel disease, Alzheimer's disease, senile dementia, parkinsons disease, multiple sclerosis, microbial infections, degenerative diseases, etc. With passage of time simple less expensive equipment will be available. At present radiant heat, dry sauna, steam baths and hot water offer excellent method of hyperthermia induction. If you are suffering from chronic diseases and AIDS, be bold, and start your own hyperthermia program at home. With little effort and minimal expense, you can obtain the benefits of hyperthermia. NO BODY CAN STOP IT.

I would rather die experimenting on my disease, than a disease experimenting, experiencing, and enjoying me and my body.

Did You Know?

Taking our body temperature began about 125 years ago. It was started by a German physician named Carl Wunderlich (1815-77) in Leipzig. At that time, the thermometers were one foot long and took 20 minute to register our body temperature.

Temperature of our body is 98.6 F. Women are 1.00 degree F. hotter after ovulation. Whereas the temperature of cat and cow is 101.5, dog 102.00, pig and sheep 102.5, rabbit 103.1, goat 103.8, chicken 107.00 (varies from 105.00 to 109.00) degree F. Scientifically, when you say " you are cool as cucumber" is a true statement. Inside temperature of a cucumber is 10 degree F. lower than the environmental temperature it is growing.

FIGURE 1: HYPERTHERMIA INDUCTION BY USING EXTRACORPOREAL CIRCULATION. THE BLOOD IS MOVED FROM THE ARTERY IN THE GROIN, HEATED BY THE HEATING COILS AND RETURNED TO THE BODY THROUGH THE VEIN.

BLOOD IS DRAWN FROM THE FEMORAL ARTERY THROUGH THE PLASTIC TUBINGS, HEATED TO 112 DEGREE FAHRENHEIT BY WATER HEATED COIL, AND RETURNED TO THE BODY THROUGH THE FEMORAL VEIN TO BRING THE BODY CORE TEMPERATURE TO 108 DEGREE F.

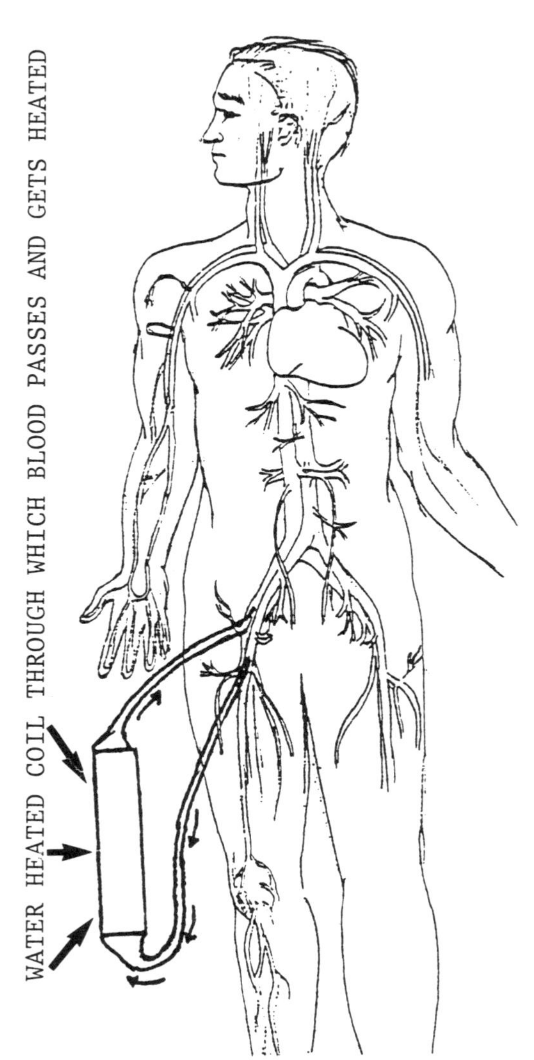

FIGURE 2: SHOWS RADIANT METHOD OF HEATING THE BODY WHICH IS SAFER COMPARED TO THE EXTRACORPOREAL METHOD.

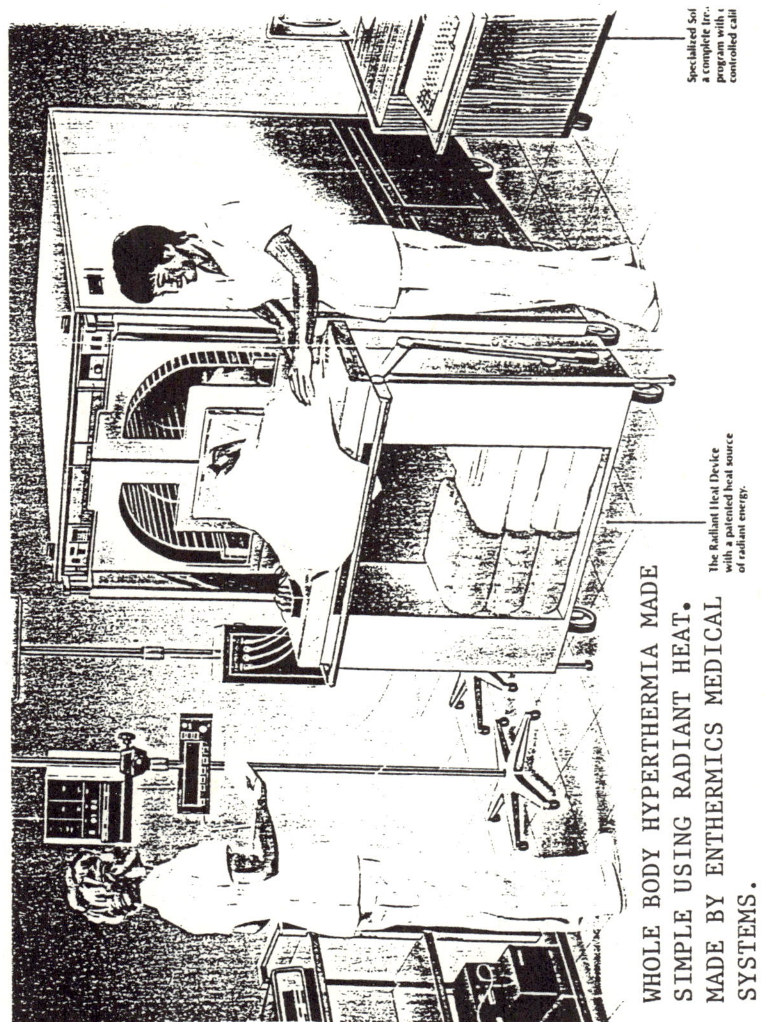

CHAPTER 2

HISTORY OF AUTOIMMUNE URINE THERAPY (AUT)

All things are possible to him who believes.
Mark 9.23

The exact origin of autoimmune urine therapy (AUT) is unknown. Autoimmune urine therapy was practiced for hundreds of years in India. In the Old and New Testaments of the Bible, there are suggestions of the healing power of autoimmune urine therapy; Proverbs 5:15 says "Drink water from your cistern and fresh water from your own well." In latin cistern means bladder.

In this book I will discuss in detail the origin of AUT, contents of urine, how AUT works, how to practice AUT, how to combine it with hyperthermia and drugs to cure or curtail many incurable chronic diseases.

The first book on autoimmune urine therapy was written by John W. Armstrong, entitled *The Water of Life* (WL). It was published in England in 1944. *The Water of Life* describes personal experiences and the diseases he claimed were cured by the autoimmune urine therapy. With the use of autoimmune urine therapy advanced cases of **tuberculosis, cancers, gangrene, nephritis, infectious diseases, malaria, allergies, asthma, paralysis, jaundice and many other acute and chronic ailments** were cured. Probably based on J. W. Armstrong's book, Mr. Raojibhai Manibhai Patel of India started the autoimmune urine therapy movement. He published the experiences of AUT in a book in the fifties called *Manava Mootra* (MM). It was translated into many Indian languages, including my mother tongue Kannada (1965). According to this book, autoimmune urine therapy cured all of the above-mentioned diseases.

Ancient Literature from India on Autoimmune Urine Therapy

In India, there exists a large body of literature that deals with this subject. *Akoota Jeevanadhori*, a book published in the Gujarthi language (1923) describes autoimmune urine therapy and its advantages. The author of this book practiced autoimmune urine therapy and lived to an exceptionally old age. He learned about autoimmune urine therapy from a priest from Norway.

There is another Sanskrit book, *Damatantra Shivambukalpa Vidhi*, written hundreds of years ago. This old tantric book was translated in the late fifties by a Sanskrit Pundit, Ramachandra B. Atavale from Bombay. It gives specific instructions about the practice of autoimmune urine therapy and its disease healing and preventing qualities. This ancient book contains a discourse between the God Shiva and his wife the Goddess Parvathi. Shiva is the Hindu god of the destruction of evil, thus making way for new and just creation. The God Shiva preaches to his wife, that drinking Shivambu (meaning urine) and applying externally cures the existing diseases. It cleanses the body and mind while creating a new vigor. Shiva instructs to drink the urine early in the morning with a clear mind, after washing face and mouth and while facing the rising sun. He instructs the urine therapist to collect the middle part of the urine in earthen or copper utensils, after discarding first and last few drops of urine.

According to this *Damatantra Shivambukalpa Vidhi* holy book, drinking urine and applying the urine on the skin for one month cleans the inside and outside of the body. In two months, urine will cleanse all the senses. In three months it will take away the worry of disease. In five months, this practice will take away worry and sadness and cure depression. Six months of AUT will make one wise and free from diseases. Continued practice of AUT for seven months will make a person physically and mentally strong. Eight months of AUT will cure KSHAYA (tuberculosis, emaciation) and KUSTA (dry disfigured skin). In 11 months, AUT will cleanse all the organs of the body and make the user youthful. Youth will be restored by two years of therapy. Practicing Shivambu (autoimmune urine therapy) for 12 years will make a person almost immortal, living a long life free from all diseases. Such a person, according to Shiva, is immune to poisonous snake bites, can resist burning, and can float on water (see Mark 16:13). This means that such a person can counteract a snake's venom with autoimmune urine therapy. Burns and wounds heal by applying the urine externally. "Resist burning" can be interpreted as curing the disease associated with high fever (fever = fire). Such a person can float on water (swim) and stay above water for many hours. A person can stay alive for a long time by using AUT without any other nourishment, if fresh water is available. Life can be sustained for three months by drinking urine with fresh water. According to ancient literature, urine also cures diseases present since birth. However, it cannot cure congenital and mechanical defects. These defects usually need modern medical care and surgery.

Lord Shiva instructs people practicing Shivambu to follow a certain regimen in their daily living. They should eat less of all foods and avoid very spicy or salty foods, eat less or no food before going to bed. They should have adequate rest, and practice moderation in sex or have no sex at all. The Yogis in India who practiced autoimmune urine therapy lived for more than 100 years and did not have gray hair or wrinkles. Besides drinking urine, Lord Shiva advocates that the urine should be rubbed on the body three times a day and three times a night. He states that the person who practices these procedures becomes very strong. Topical application opens all the pores of the skin. The heart is cleansed along with all other organs and their connections (ducts) and their openings. It makes them function properly. Breathing urine through the nose will heal all the ailments of the respiratory tract (nose, larynx, lungs, pharynx) and stomach. Finally, Shiva says, "My dear Parvathi, I have described the procedures of urine therapy and its benefits, keep it to yourself." It should be told only to those who can practice and accept (*Manavamootra Malamootra*, 1965).

Ancient Jain literature from India, such as *Bhadrabhavu in Vyavahara Sutra* also contains instructions about urine therapy. Ayurvedic (Indian medical system) books by Sushutra, Haritha, Bhavaprakasha, Yogaratnakara, and Vrudhavagh Bhatta (*Astranga*) contain instructions on the usefulness of urine therapy (*Manavamootra Malamootra*, 1965). Today, in many villages of India, cattle and human urine is given to drink as a remedy for various ailments. In Tibet many Llamas (Buddhist priests) practiced urine therapy in their daily lives. Many of the Llamas practicing urine therapy live for more than 150 years. They are without any diseases and traveled great stretches of desert and land by foot. Maurice Wilson, who attempted to climb Mount Everest before Tenzing Norgay and Edmund Hillary in 1953, practiced autoimmune urine therapy (both drinking and external application). According to Wilson, AUT gave him stamina and strength, and protected him against colds, bronchitis, and pneumonia. He learned about autoimmune urine therapy by associating with Llamas and Yogis of Tibet and Nepal.

Experiences of People Stranded without Food and Water

There are reports of people stranded in shipwrecks, boats, deserts, forests, and mountains that had exhausted all of their food and water. They sustained life by drinking their own urine until help arrived. A recent example is the survival of nearly 50 (out of more than 100) South Vietnam people fleeing the communist rule by boat. They were trapped in the boat for many days. They survived by cannibalism and urine drinking after exhausting all of their food and fresh water. In July 1990, the island of Philippines had a big earth quake in which thousands of people died. The last survivor was pulled out of a hotel rubble alive and healthy 14 days after the quake. He gave a statement that he survived by drinking his own urine and rain water. The other two with him died because they did not drink urine and water.

Old English Literature on Autoimmune urine therapy

Christian missionaries in Africa and India gave some medicine (both herbal, modern, and homeopathic) along with urine to heal the sick. They obtained urine specimens on the pretext of testing for diseases. As a child, I was told to put urine on injury on my legs or hands. I did accordingly, and the wounds would heal without any infections. *Salmon's English Physicians* (1865), an English book, describes urine as the serum or watery part of the blood. The blood serum is diverted by emulgent arteries and veins of the kidneys, where it is separated, fermented, and concentrated into urine. It has dissolving, cleansing, and purifying properties, and prevents putrefaction. Drinking urine, protects against the obstruction of the liver, spleen, and gallbladder and organized dropsy, jaundice, menstruation disorders, plagues, and high fevers. It is an excellent remedy for tremors, Parkinson's disease, numbness, and palsy. The volatile salts of urine are powerful absorbers of acids that destroy the very root of most diseases in the human body. These volatile salts open all obstructions of the urinary tract, mesentery, and the womb. Urine purifies the blood, and cures cachexia, rheumatism, hypochondriacs, epilepsy, vertigo, apoplexy, convulsions, lethargies, migraine, lameness, numbness, loss of use of the limbs, atrophies, and colds, and diseases of the nerves, joints, etc. Urine dissolves coagulations and opens obstructions of the kidney. It breaks and expels renal stones. It is a specific remedy for dysuria, ischuria, and obstruction of the urinary flow. Urine applied externally cleans and softens the skin. It disinfects common wounds and wounds caused by poisonous weapons. Its application also cures dandruff and scuff, and cools the heat of fever.

In the last century, a popular book was published in English, entitled *One Thousand Notable Things*, in which autoimmune urine therapy was described as one of the most important treatments. According to this book, drinking urine every morning for nine days will cure scurvy, jaundice, swelling, and make the body light and the mind cheerful. Urine is a universal remedy for distemper, inward and outward. Washing the ear with urine will heal ear ailments, cures deafness, and stops the ringing in the ear. Washing the eyes with urine will cure sore eyes and clear and strengthen the sight. Urine application cures chapped, rough hands. Urine applied to an itching site takes away the itching, makes the joints limber, and makes the wound heal faster. Washing the anorectal area (fundament) with urine is a good protection against hemorrhoids and other sores.

Mr. Armstrong's book describes another urine therapy case in which Mr. W. H. Baxter of Leeds drank urine and lived to a very old age. He claimed that drinking three tumblers full of urine a day acted as prophylaxis against disease and cured many ailments. He cured a cancerous growth by applying his own urine compressors and by drinking it. He used it externally on his eyes and improved his vision, and applied it on his face after shaving to improve his complexion. He advocated its external use for wounds, swelling, and boils. He claimed urine to be an excellent laxative. My own personal experience has shown that it is an excellent laxative.

Urine Therapy in Persia and Egypt

In the 18th Century, a Parisian dentist, Fauchard, advocated washing the mouth and cleansing the teeth with urine. It made the mouth clean, the teeth strong, and relieved tooth ache (*Devils Drugs and Doctors*, 1928, p. 328). Early Egyptian physicians used the urine of a faithful wife as effective treatment for sore eyes (*Devils Drugs and Doctors*, page 336). Trachoma, also known as Egyptian conjunctivitis is a chronic contagious form of conjunctivitis. It affects 400 million people, mostly in Africa and Asia. It is caused by a strain of Chlamydia trachomatous, an organism related to bacteria and rickettsia. It is treated by the local application of erythromycin and tetracycline. An estimated 20 million people have become blind because of trachoma. With urine application, blindness due to trachoma can be prevented if modern medical treatment is not available.

Gypsies and Urine Therapy

Besides human urine, bovine urine (urine from cow or a bull) has curative power, too. A Dorset farmer (U.K.), just before the turn of the century, drank four pints of cow's urine everyday for 60 years. He started this habit at the age of 20 and had never become ill since that time. His posture was straight in spite of his old age. This farmer obtained the secret of autoimmune urine therapy from a gypsy while suffering from throat and chest ailments. Gypsies originated in India hundreds of years ago. Autoimmune urine therapy, which gypsies continue to practice even now, was widespread in India. Indians designate the cow and bull as holy animals. Besides the disease healing qualities of their urine, cows provide milk for children and dung for fertilizer. Cows are easy to tame and maintain, and the bulls are used in agriculture. Gradually, holiness was bestowed on them to prevent their slaughtering for food. I do believe cow's urine does heal. Since cattle urine is genetically different--its food habits are different--its urine constituents are also different from that of humans. The diseases cows suffer are also different. Thus antigen and antibodies produced are of a different nature. Therefore, auto (self, own) autoimmune urine therapy is far superior to using cow's urine. Further discussion of this subject read Chapter 12.

The Bible and Urine Therapy

The Bible has many quotes about holy drinks and their healing power. I interpret the holy water, streams, and drinks as urine. Plain water, no matter where it comes from, how much it is blessed, and by whom it is blessed, has no disease healing qualities. It is the urine that has the healing qualities. Genesis 1:2 says, "The Spirit of God was moving over the water." This can be interpreted as that both fresh water and urine contain the Spirit of God and have satisfying and healing power. Psalms 46:4 says, "There is a river whose streams make glad the city of God, the holy dwelling places of the most high." The river refers to the body fluids, which come out in a stream as urine. The human body, especially the heart, is the dwelling place of God, Supreme Spirit, Soul, or Holy Ghost. "The city of God is made glad" means the body is purified and made disease free. Psalms 23:2 says, "He leadeth me beside still waters; He restoreth my soul." This can be interpreted as, those who guide the sick and afflicted to autoimmune urine therapy (still water) can restore their health and spirit back to normal.

Ecclesiastes 31:6, 7, 8, and 9 says, "Give strong drink to him who is perishing and wine to him whose life is bitter. Let him drink and forget his poverty and remember his trouble no more. Open the mouth for the drink for the rights of all unfortunate. Open your mouth, judge righteously and defend the right of the afflicted and needy." There are two types of drink recommended by the author of Ecclesiastes: One is strong drink meaning urine, and the other is wine. The strong drink (urine) is good for the poor and unfortunate (sick) because it costs nothing and makes ailments go away. The last paragraph (31:9) clearly tells that those who prescribe this therapy should know how to use it (judge righteously).

John 4:10 says, "If you know the gift of God and who it is who says to you, Give me drink, you would have asked him and he would have given you living water." When one asks God for a drink, he gives him living water. The fresh water is the water of life no doubt, but it is not living water. Urine is the living water, containing all the constituents of the body and more. Revelations 22:17 says, "Let the one who wishes take the water of life without cost." The only water available without cost is urine. In ancient times, people paid money to use well water.

Mark 16:16, 17, and 18 says, "He who believes and has been baptized shall be saved; but he who has disbelieved shall be condemned. They will cast out demons and they will speak with a new tongue. They will pick up serpents and if they drink poison, it shall not hurt them; they will lay their hands on the sick and they will recover." These verses are interpreted differently by different religious groups and Bible scholars. I believe this scripture meant that, if one believes in autoimmune urine therapy and practices it, the sick will be saved and mental sickness will be healed (cast out demons). If they cannot speak (due to nervous system diseases including strokes), through autoimmune urine therapy they will speak again (speak with a new tongue). Autoimmune urine therapy protects against poisonous snake and insect bites. It protects those who drink poison (Mark 16:18). Such cases of healing by autoimmune urine therapy are reported in India. When Mark (16:18) says that those who believe in the practice of autoimmune urine therapy (believe in me and baptism) can convince the sick to do the same (lay hands on the sick), such sick people will be healed. Many healing ministers take this passage from the Bible. They have been healing people afflicted with birth defects, deafness, cancers, backaches, and every disease known to the world. We know that these ministers cannot cure all the ailments they claim. But we have no doubt that those with hope, love, faith, and positive feelings do help in healing some diseases and accelerate recovery. The healing ministers can bring a positive feeling within the sick and a hope for a miraculous cure. Chapter 20 contains more details on the healing power of a positive thinker.

There is a sect of Christians in Tennessee and other places who dance with poisonous snakes on their bodies and hands as a part of a religious ceremony. They believe that the snake bite will not kill them if they handle the snake in the name of the Lord (Mark 16:18). Unfortunately many of these participants have died of snake bites. We know that cancers do disappear and some diseases subside without any explanation. This phenomenon is explained on the basis of the body's immune defense mechanisms gaining control over the disease processes. Blessing by healing ministers can only help such phenomenon. Positive thinking can also stimulate the brain to produce morphine like substances called endorphins. Hyperthermia also increases endorphines. Endorphins reduce muscle and joint pains. There is evidence to support the theory that positive thinking can enhance the immune system in curing deadly diseases, such as cancers (psychoneuro-immunology, visualization therapy; see Chapter 20).

Faith Healing - As an Extension of AUT

There is a sect of Christian Scientists in the U.S.A. who practice praying for all kinds of illness. They believe in spiritual healing. The praying for healing is guided by spiritual practitioners. Many patients have lost their life by following this method of treatment. A seven year old diabetic child from Florida, a small boy suffering from meningitis in Iowa, and a child with intestinal obstruction in Boston died as a result of this praying therapy. The parents of one such child were convicted of third degree murder for not rendering proper medical care. I believe practicing spiritual healing along with autoimmune urine therapy will heal most diseases. These Christian Scientists have interpreted the Bible incorrectly and practiced incomplete therapy.

Diseases such as bowel obstructions, intestinal perforations, broken bones, meningitis, bleeding, etc., have to be surgically and medically treated, besides praying and autoimmune urine therapy. The Bible says, "If thy hand or thy foot offends thee, cut them off . . . if thine eye offend thee, pluck it out and cast it from thee (Matthew 18: 8-9)." These verses mean that any diseased part of the body should be removed so that the whole body does not suffer with pain and may even lead to death (cast into fire). Micro-organisms also cause pain and suffering. Praying alone will not help. The ailment needs to be eradicated by proper therapy besides praying. Many of the Jehovah's Witnesses sect of Christians refuse to receive blood when they are bleeding and die as result of it. I do not believe God intended this approach to life, sickness and death. Death resulting from praying to cure a diseases without proper medical treatment and AUT is a form of homicide. Many diseases we suffer are self limiting. They disappear without any intervention with a lapse of time. That does not mean healing was achieved due to prayer. There is no doubt that it can be combined with AUT and hyperthermia to enhance the healing processes.

It is clear from the above discussion, that autoimmune urine therapy has been in practice for many thousands of years all over the world. Urine therapy alone or combining it with hyperthermia, drugs, surgery, radiation etc. can cure or curtail many diseases. It costs nothing and has no adverse effects on the body. **URINE IS THE WATER WITH LIFE AND WATER OF LIFE.**

CHAPTER 3

MR. J. W. ARMSTRONG'S EXPERIENCE

Fortunate is the person who has developed the self control to steer a straight course towards his objective.
Napoleon Hill

The first modern book on autoimmune urine therapy, *The Water of Life*, was written by J. W. Armstrong of England (1944). Armstrong was thirty-four years old when he went to enlist in the British Army during World War I. He was examined by four army doctors and diagnosed as a case of tuberculosis of the lungs and rejected for army enlistment. A physician treated him by prescribing fresh air, sunshine, and a nourishing diet. By this method of treatment, he gained 25 pounds in one year. However, he remained unhappy and consulted a second physician. He confirmed the diagnosis of tuberculosis of both lungs and added more sugars and starches to his diet. This diet resulted in diabetes. He was put on five days starvation, followed by two days of snacking. Gradually he became very ill and weak.

After two years of medical treatment, he lost faith in physicians and began experimenting with autoimmune urine therapy. He cites the Bible, Proverbs 5:15, "Drink water out of thine own cistern," and states that this means drink urine from the bladder. Besides the Bible quote, I believe he came to know about autoimmune urine (AUT) therapy from other people who had tried and cured serious diseases with it. He fasted for 45 days and drank all of his urine and tap water. He used part of his urine to rub on the skin over his entire body. At the end of the therapy, he states that his disease was gone and he felt like a new man, weighing 140 pounds, with a vigorous body, and looking younger than his age (36). He broke 45 day fast by eating raw beef and had an excellent appetite. He is not specific about his future practice of AUT. It appears that he drank all the urine, every drop of it, every day, and ate a small meal. It seems that he continued this practice until his death at the age of 63. He never suffered again from any minor or major ailments. He eventually developed heart problems as a result of weight lifting and strenuous exercise and died suddenly. I presume he died of aortic valve disease (regurgitation and left ventricular hypertrophy) caused by heavy weight lifting.

From his personal experience, Armstrong started advocating and advising autoimmune urine therapy to cure various diseases. He wrote the monograph, *The Water of Life* based on his AUT experience. He reports **curing gangrene, malaria, cancers (various kinds), heart disease, breast cancers, several kinds of skin conditions, diabetes, kidney disease, jaundice, high blood pressure, fevers of unknown origin, leukemia, orchitis (infection of the testes), many types of infectious diseases, venereal disease, burns, enuresis nocturia (bed wetting), menstrual trouble, bronchial asthma, prostrate trouble, obesity, warts, skin rashes, premature aging, paralysis, loss of memory, baldness, glaucoma, cataract, arthritis, insect bites (bee sting), anemia, tuberculosis, mucous colitis, psoriasis, lupus, pyorrhea (gum disease), thyroid conditions, pneumonia, appendicitis, pleurisy, rheumatism, common cold, etc.** Armstrong makes sarcastic comments on modern medicine. There are many misquotes about the etiology of various diseases in his book. These mistakes were made due to a lack of proper medical background and some prejudice.

CHAPTER 4

EXPERIENCES IN INDIA

The preservation of health is a duty
Herbert Spencer

Shivambukalpa Vidhi, a tantric Sanskrit book written hundreds of years ago, contains complete instructions on autoimmune urine therapy (AUT). Autoimmune urine therapy is described in many ancient Hindu religious and medical books. It is practiced even now by the Yogis of India and the Llamas of Tibet. The practice of autoimmune urine therapy AUT) was almost forgotten in India until R. M. Patel reintroduced it. He probably came to know about autoimmune urine therapy by reading J. W. Armstrong's book, *The Water of Life*, (WL) and then used it on himself. He prescribed and supervised AUT on many people. Based on his and other people's experiences, he published a book in the Gujarathi language in the fifties, *Manava Mootra Swamootra* (MM). Autoimmune urine therapy in India is popular in Gujarath, Bombay, and Karnataka states. This therapy is prescribed and promoted by those who have been successful in treating their own diseases.

The following are a few examples of ailments that are claimed to have been cured by autoimmune urine therapy in India: **allergic conditions, eczema, psoriasis, tuberculosis, malaria, infectious diseases, jaundice, heart disease, arthritis, peptic ulcers, cancers, leukemia, Hodgkin's disease, nephritis, weakness, colitis, appendicitis, diabetes, high blood pressure, ear aches, chronic ulcers, stroke, old age, influenza, pneumonia, leprosy, lupus, snake bites, insect bites, hair loss, dandruff, gangrene, teeth problems, and many other health problems.** Followers of this therapy claim that no matter what the disease or how it came about, Shivambu, meaning drinking your own urine, will cure all ailments. They do not give the exact reason of how or why the autoimmune urine therapy works. It is believed to act by removing wastes and toxins from the body and stimulating the immune system. There are no hospitals where patients are admitted and treated with autoimmune urine therapy. Therefore, drinking urine for various diseases and documenting how it works in a hospital setting is needed. Since the death of J. W. Armstrong, the autoimmune urine therapy movement has come to a stand still in England. In India there are thousands of followers who practice autoimmune urine therapy on a daily basis. These include the ex-Chief Minister of India, M. Desai and myself.

Autoimmune Urine Therapy Experience's of the Prime Minister of India

The former Prime Minister of India, Morarji Desai, who is 81 years old, works 12 hours a day. He travels incessantly around India and conducts business well. The secret of his youthful vim is derived from the regimen he follows: daily doses of carrot and apple juice, milk, yogurt, honey, fresh fruits, nuts, dates, five cloves of raw garlic, and consumption of a glass of morning urine. He has been drinking a glass of morning urine since 1971. He cured his brother of tuberculosis with autoimmune urine therapy. He declares that "urine is the water of life. It is very good for you and it is even free" (*Time*, October 22, 1977, p. 58). Even as I write this book, former Prime Minister Desai is alive and healthy at the age of 95. He has practiced autoimmune urine therapy for eighteen years. In a public speech given in Ahamadabad, India, he stressed the need for auto autoimmune urine therapy for millions of poor who could not afford costly medicines. Speaking at the auto autoimmune urine therapy conference organized at the Gujarath Vidyapeeth, he states that the secret of his sound health and mental ability has been the result of years of practicing autoimmune urine therapy. Desai claimed that the regular dose of urine cured his physical ailments and mental disorders (*News India*, October 23, 1987, p. 13).

Experiences in Jail

Narabhai Panter, from Bombay was imprisoned in 1933 at the age of 17 for participating in India's independence movement. He went on a hunger strike for five days as a protest. For this act, he was tied to a pole and lashed 15 times. There were bruises and lacerations on his body measuring 8 inches by 1 inch. In the jail at that time there was a notorious criminal in jail named Dawaud Ghani. He took pity on this young man and told him to drink urine and to apply it on his wounds. Panter followed these instructions and was completely healed within four days. In 1942, he was jailed again and went on a hunger strike. On the 16th day of hunger, his urine output decreased to trickles and then to a few drops a day. He feared kidney failure and remembering Ghani's advise, started drinking all the urine he produced. This resulted in increased urine production, and his kidneys resumed normal functioning. When Panter was in the Erode Jail, many of the prisoners suffered from yellow jaundice. He treated them successfully with autoimmune urine therapy (MM, p. 260).

Healing Power of the Ganges River Water

Water from the Ganges River in North India is claimed to have healing properties. According to Armstrong, this healing property is due to the presence of traces of urine. People, while bathing, urinate in the water and drink the water also. On analysis, the Ganges water contains minute traces of urine. I doubt very much that such small traces of urine in billions of gallons of water can have the healing properties that are claimed. It is likely that the healing power of the Ganges water, attributed by many, is due to placebo effects, positive suggestion, belief, and faith.

CHAPTER 5

MY EXPERIENCE WITH AUTOIMMUNE URINE THERAPY AND HYPERTHERMIA

Experiments and experiences are great teachers.
T.R. Shantha

No wild enthusiast ever yet could rest until
half mankind were like himself possessed.
Cowper

Background

I came to the United States from India in 1960 on a fellowship to the Emory University School of Medicine to study for a Ph.D in basic sciences. Before that, I had M.D. degree (M.B.B.S. at R. G. Kar Medical College, India) from the University of Calcutta (1958). After that I was appointed as an assistant surgeon in the S.D.S. Sanitarium (Bangalore). I was involved in the treatment of tuberculosis patients and assisting in thoracic surgery. Then I worked in The Victoria Hospital, Bangalore (India), in the E.N.T. and Cardiology departments. Finally I was appointed as a lecturer in the Department of Anatomy, Bangalore Medical College before coming to the United States.

I started my research at the Emory University Anatomy Department on the membranes of the peripheral nerves. My first research paper was published by the Rockefeller Institute's *The Journal of Cell Biology* in 1962. I obtained Ph.D. in 1962 and continued to do research and teach. So far I have published more than 100 research papers in internationally known research journals and 5 books. Seven of my articles were published in the distinguished British journal *Nature*.

Back to My Motherland

In 1963 I heard from India that my beloved mother was suffering from cancer of the cervix. I was unable to go back to India immediately because of visa problems. My mother died a few weeks prior to my arrival in 1965. She was treated with radiation, homeopathic, and local folklore therapies. I stayed in India for three months and completed the final religious rites of my mother's demise. I returned to Emory University and continued to work in the Anatomy Department as Associate Professor.

Subsequently, I have visited India 4 more times. My father also passed away in 1977. A girls high school was build in my father and mother's name at Hosadurga, close to my birth place (Janthikolalu and Devigere) in India **(Totada Ramaiah, Gowramma Memorial Girls High School)**. We provided major funding for the construction of this building. It provides excellent class room facilities for 300 girls. It was officially opened by Hon. Chief Minister of Karnataka, Mr.S.R. Bommaiah on 13th September of 1988. My son, Devendra, a final year medical student in JJM medical college, attended the opening ceremony. My wife Victoria Kay, my children Devendra, Usha and Anand helped me immensely in this project.

Questioned About Urine Therapy During My Visits to India

It was during my visits to India, I was asked for my opinion on urine therapy. During my childhood I was told to apply urine on any injury and skin conditions which I did and got cured. I had forgotten about it completely. Autoimmune urine therapy has been in practice in various parts of the world, both East and West. No research scientist has written about it and explained on scientific basis how the autoimmune urine therapy (AUT) cures diseases. J. W. Armstrong and R. J. Patel published books describing urine therapy cures. These men were nonmedical authors and explained their experiences. I obtained *The Water of Life* (1944) by ordering it through the

Emory University Bookstore in 1965. I obtained the treatise on autoimmune urine therapy, written by R. M. Patel translated in Kannada (*Manavamootra and Malamootra*, 1965 edition) from India. Both these books contain numerous cases of complete cures of various infectious diseases, psoriasis, jaundice, heart disease, kidney disease, cancer, leukemia, tuberculosis, eczema, etc.

As I read both the books, it was apparent to me, that there was something to autoimmune urine therapy, but there was hardly any scientific explanation of why and how autoimmune urine therapy works. There were many misconceptions quoted in these books about the etiology of various diseases. There was a lot of sarcasm expressed against modern physicians. In spite of these deficiencies, these two books do show to the medical community how modern medicine has neglected such a simple inexpensive remedy. We have also failed to investigate scientifically the reasons behind autoimmune urine therapy cures of various diseases.

Urine Freeze drying Experiments at The Yerkes Regional Primate Research Center

In latter part of 1965, I was moved to the Yerkes Regional Primate Research Center of Emory University (with Professor G. H. Bourne who died in July 19, 1988, at the age of 78), Atlanta, Georgia, as the Director of Neurohistochemistry and Associate Professor of Ophthalmology. I was conducting pure basic research in neurohistochemistry, neuroanatomy, and the histology of the primate nervous system and eye. Urine therapy was still on my mind. I thought, instead of drinking the whole urine, why not freeze dry the urine. The solid material after this processes can be placed in gelatin capsules, which can be easily swallowed without any inhibition. I obtained a freeze drying machine from the Ophthalmic Laboratory (courtesy of Drs. M. Waitzman and Richard Jackson) at Emory University and attempted to freeze dry urine. It took more than 24 hours to freeze dry a glass of urine and only a few grams of dried material was obtained. I began to realize that this process was lengthy, expensive, and impractical. I abandoned my experiments on urine freeze drying.

I gave a copy of the autoimmune urine therapy book to the veterinarian in Yerkes Primate Research Center. We discussed the prospect of starting a autoimmune urine therapy project for canine cancer (lymphosarcoma). After reading the book by J. W. Armstrong, he returned it and wrote me, "After reading this book and thinking about your proposed urine therapy for canine lymphosarcoma, I would like to back down from what we discussed previously. I think the book is completely beyond reason and without any scientific basis. I became greatly disturbed by reading this book because of the constant downgrading of the medical profession by Armstrong. We can discuss this in more detail if you like," signed Dr. M (1965). After this letter, I completely dropped the project until I encountered the case of diffuse, extensive, atherosclerotic coronary artery disease I describe below.

Moving to Clinical Practice

In 1968, due to many personal and financial commitments, I returned to clinical medicine. I completed anesthesiology residency program at the Emory University School of Medicine. At that time I won first prize in resident research paper contest for two consecutive years. I was appointed as an associate professor in the Department of Anesthesiology at the Emory University School of Medicine. In 1973 I entered a private practice in anesthesiology at the Georgia Baptist Medical Center in Atlanta and Columbus Medical Center. In 1989 I was appointed as visiting professor in JJM Medical College in Davanagere, Karnataka, India.

Experiment on a Coronary Artery Disease Patient

In 1974 I heard my friend (a mathematics professor at the University of North Carolina in Charlotte) was suffering from severe coronary artery disease. A Cardiologist performed an angiogram and found severe atherosclerosis of all the coronary arteries, including obstruction of the right coronary artery (RCA) and left anterior descending branch (LAD). The circumflex artery was 80% occluded. The cardiologist corresponded with me and stated in the letter, "I do not understand how this man is living." The heart surgeon indicated to me that my friend might not survive an open heart procedure (coronary artery bypass graft surgery) because of the severity of the disease.

I had two books in the Kannada language on urine therapy and showed my friend that autoimmune urine therapy could help him. He was hesitant to drink his urine. I finally convinced him to come to Atlanta to my home. I took a leave from work for a week and began fasting and drinking urine with him every day for a week. We broke the fast with a small meal. He felt better, lost weight, looked great, and could walk a longer distance without much chest pain. He went to India and walked for hours in the hot sun over-stressing his heart. He died in a nursing home on August 8, 1986, of congestive heart failure. However, he had lived ten years with severe heart disease, when originally his cardiologist had given him only three months to live.

Experimentation on My Friends and Myself on Poison Ivy, Skin Conditions, Burns, Herpes, Keratitis (eye), Asthma, Dandruff, Hair Loss etc.

I decided to continue the practice of autoimmune urine therapy on myself, my family and friend and study the effects. According to the two published monographs, fresh and old urine is said to be an excellent remedy when applied and gently massaged two to three times a day for chapped hands, blisters, sores, stings, barber rash, allergic conditions, skin eruptions such as herpes, and skin irritation caused by contact with allergic or toxic materials or plants such as poison ivy. My wife, Victoria, was working in our back yard preparing the ground for spring planting. She came in contact with a poison ivy plant and developed redness, itching, and blisters. She used creams, local anesthetic sprays and steroid ointments without any relief. At my insistence, she began applying urine using cotton swabs on seventeen areas (one to two inches in diameter) of skin on her legs and hands. She applied urine three to four times a day starting in the mornings for five days. She was relieved of itching within an hour. The redness, itching and blisters disappeared. No one in the hospital where she works complained of smelling urine. I have advocated this to many nurses and friends for poison ivy, burns, rashes and insect bites. They have used this therapy with success.

I developed a peculiar skin condition in 1965. I developed small button sized areas of hyper-pigmentation (dark areas) with scaling, dryness, and itching. They were located mainly on my thighs, buttocks, the upper arms area, and the back side of my chest. I consulted three physicians, one of them a Professor of Dermatology at the university where I worked. Two skin biopsies were taken, stained, and examined under a microscope to find the true nature of the disease. Still they could not diagnose the disease. All three dermatologists I consulted recommended topical application of steroid (cortisone) ointment on the lesions. There were hundreds of such spots appearing and disappearing. I did use skin steroid ointment which gave only temporary relief. Because of the dangers of steroid therapy, I discontinued its use. I started drinking morning urine every day, beginning January 1, 1987. My skin condition started to improve. I started using jacuzzi set at 105°F (mild hyperthermia) almost every other day. The skin conditions started improving much faster. The number of rashes appearing in crops also lessened. I also applied old and new urine on these spots rubbing the urine in well. Many spots on my trunk, buttocks, and thighs have disappeared. I do believe that the hyperthermia and AUT have synergistic effect in healing the chronic conditions.

In 1968 I had developed an allergy, which would last the entire month of April every year. I suffered from itching and watering of the eyes and nose, redness of my eyes, a raw feeling in my pharynx and soft palate, and bronchial asthma attacks which were severe at night. I had to take many antibiotics, antihistamines, and bronchodilator drugs for four to five weeks during these attacks every year. All these drugs caused drowsiness and increased my heart rate. Many nights, I could not sleep due to asthmatic attacks (bronchospasm), resulting in difficulty in exhaling air (expiratory wheezes). In 1982, I was attending a cooking class in place of my wife. The cooking instructor, while talking about garlic, mentioned that she was allergic to support hose. She got cured from her allergy by taking garlic tablets (obtained from the health food stores). I took that suggestion and started taking garlic tablets every two to four hours during the spring allergy season (April). This reduced my allergy. The only drawback was that sometimes I had to take 15-18 tablets a day. The effect lasted only two to four hours, and I had to get up in the middle of the night to take garlic tablets.

Since I started drinking morning urine every day, the attacks of allergy and allergic bronchial asthma, which would appear in April, are considerably reduced (95% relief), and I only have to take two to four garlic tablets a day. This year (1990) my allergic condition is 98% relieved. I took a total of twelve garlic tablets for the whole season. I also inhaled morning urine through my nose and instilled it in my eyes and nose with the use of a dropper 2-3 times a day. I have hardly experienced any itching, tearing, or postnasal drip. It appears by my personal experience that only small doses of drugs are need to cure or curtail a disease during urine therapy, hyperthermia and dry sauna treatment. My allergy and skin condition is almost cured. I also suffered from severe dandruff and loss of hair. Applying urine on my scalp has stopped the hair loss and reduced the dandruff.

A patient from Americus, Georgia, suffered from keratitis of both eyes for years. She was treated with many expensive drugs for months without any relief. On my wife's insistence she applied urine eye drops 3-4 times a day. She experienced complete relief within a week and does not have to spend any money on drugs. One of our family friends' mother and her friend close to 80 years old suffered from painful herpes zoster of the chest wall. Modern medication had very little effect. Application of morning urine on the herpes lesions 3 to 4 times a day completely relieved the pain, and the spots were dried out completely.

These experiences show that autoimmune urine therapy can certainly cure many curable and incurable diseases at no cost. The knowledge of autoimmune urine therapy and hyperthermia can be of immense value and even lifesaving, especially when medical help is not available or does not work.

My Experience in Hyperthermia

I participated in hyperthermia induction in advanced cancers to prolong the life and to cure the disease in 1981. Hyperthermia was induced by using the extracorporeal method. I developed the protocol for monitoring, fluid and electrolyte balance, maintaining the vital signs and proper anesthetic technique. This protocol was followed in an Atlanta hospital to induce hyperthermia in AIDS patients. We treated more than half dozen cases using this method. Hyperthermia as I described in chapter 1, using extracorporeal method should not be used. It is dangerous, life threatening, expensive, and involves too many physicians and nursing personnel. Simpler methods are available and should be tried before adopting this therapy. I have experimented with heat therapy using heated jacuzzi and hot tubs to induce mild skin hyperthermia and wet towels heated in the micro wave ovens or rinsed in hot water for local hyperthermia with good results. Most of the skin infections, boils, eye lid infections, lymph node enlargements, swelling after intramuscular injections etc. responded to local hyperthermia.

Hyperthermia is the most neglected field of medicine. Besides cancer, it can be adopted for rabies, leprosy, tuberculosis, heart and blood vessel, and nervous system diseases, etc. I came across practice of hyperthermia to treat pneumonia in our village in forties. Pneumococcal pneumonia claimed many lives before antibiotics were available. The patients of pneumonia were put under a thick blanket and were made to inhale hot steam from boiling water. Many of the patients did get better. I am sure the villagers did not know that the heat from the steam they were inhaling was killing the microbes and unplugging the clogged lungs.

CHAPTER 6

PROPONENTS AND OPPONENTS OF AUTOIMMUNE URINE THERAPY (AUT) AND HYPERTHERMIA

Any party which takes credit for the rain must not be surprised if its opponents blame it for the drought.
D.W.Morrow

A great many people think they are thinking when they are really rearranging their prejudices and superstition.
Edward R. Marrow

There are autoimmune urine therapy (AUT) followers in England and India who vehemently believe that drinking one's own urine can cure all diseases. They claim that one does not have to diagnose or know anything about the disease. The minute one becomes ill, if one begins the autoimmune urine therapy, the disease will disappear. The continued practice of daily autoimmune urine therapy along with external application to the skin will make a person disease free and youthful, with skin like a baby and able to live happily to an old age. The late J. W. Armstrong, an ardent proponent of AUT, did not believe that the doctors were ignoramuses. On the contrary, he states, "They cannot see the wood of truth for the tree of learning." The same accusations are made by many physicians who accuse urine therapists as believers in something without any scientific basis. How can it be of such importance to take back into the body that which the body is discarding? The stigma against urine ingestion is simply a cultural stigma.

Urine is considered an excreta that should not be touched. Humans are not born with religion but adopt the faith into which they are born as they grow up. The faith one believes usually depends upon our parents. So it is with the practice of autoimmune urine therapy. Drinking urine depends on how one is brought up. It is like being a vegetarian or a non-vegetarian. Among Hindu's in India, though the families may belong to the Hindu religion, some members eat meat and others do not. If one is born to a family whose members eat meat, one will be a non-vegetarian Hindu and vice versa. The customs in the family and society affect one's practices. The same is true of autoimmune urine therapy. My family and friends accepts autoimmune urine therapy because, I make certain they all observe my practice.

Many mistakes made by J.W. Armstrong and R. M. Patel regarding the causation and interpretation of various diseases, have added to the autoimmune urine therapy controversy. This provokes the medical profession to oppose autoimmune urine therapy to a greater extent. Repeated sarcastic remarks are made regarding the greed of doctors, causes of diseases, and why they do not want to include autoimmune urine therapy into their practice. For example, J. W. Armstrong writes in his book (*The Water of Life*) "What after all is syphilis? It is simply the result of a poison which is absorbed into the body and hence the rational treatment is to get that poison out of the body." It is well known that the syphilis is not caused by a poison but by a spirochete called *Treponema pallidum*. He also mis-states that Bright's disease (kidney disease) is caused by a lack of phosphates of calcium (page 31) and that lupus is caused by *Tubercle bacilli* (page 83), etc. According to Ayurvedic medicine, the human body is made up of five basic elements: earth, water, fire, air, and the sky. As long as these are in harmony, one has perfect health, and an imbalance will cause diseases. Historically, Western medicine may not accept this concept.

Yet, according to evolution, we are nothing but a collection of 75 trillion cells evolved from the sea and moved on to the beaches and land mass. Oxygen in the air sustains life, the sky provides the required water, and the earth provides life-sustaining environment and food. Fire, meaning the sun, gives the energy and the heat necessary to maintain life and grow food. The origin of disease can be caused by organisms from the earth, water, air (sky), and heat (chemical and physical factors). These elements do play a role in origin of diseases.

Supporters of autoimmune urine therapy claim that the charges of their detractor's stem from the ignorance of natural principles and deep rooted prejudice, along with the vested interest in maintaining the current medical system. Doctors and drug companies may loose their livelihood if AUT becomes a cure-all medicine. Autoimmune urine therapy advocates proclaim that the Shivambu (auto or self autoimmune urine therapy) does not require the assistance or diagnosis of doctors and it is even free. One only has to drink it to get rid of all maladies.

Can the Cures Claimed by the AUT Proponents Be Due to the Placebo Effect?

Renal physiologists, nephrologist, and traditional medical professionals look down on autoimmune urine therapy. They believe that urine contains waste products. If they are not eliminated, these waste products will lead to sickness and death (uremia). They claim that the production of urine fulfills two functions: (1) to eliminate waste products of the normal life process, and (2) to maintain a chemical balance in the body. The opponents of autoimmune urine therapy remark that it makes no sense to take back the very substance the kidneys have expelled. They also state that the body never excretes the substances it needs (which is not true). These physicians suspect cures attributed to autoimmune urine therapy are merely a placebo effect. Placebo, a remedy regardless of its nature, works because of the patients psychological belief in its efficacy. They claim that cures obtained through autoimmune urine therapy are due to strong auto suggestion rather than to the therapeutic (curative) properties present in the urine itself. Placebo work by relieving the patient of his psychosomatic symptoms. As you read, it will become clear to you that it does not cure by a placebo effect. It has healing properties.

Can AUT Cause Poisoning (Uremia)?

Many medical people believe drinking urine will cause urine poisoning. This can result in death. Death is said to be caused by the accumulation of toxic products, especially urea-related compounds. Nearly 250 nephrologists gathered in 1978 at the Downstate Medical Center in Brooklyn, N.Y., to discuss the non-dialytic management of uremia. Their final conclusion was that uremia remains a riddle wrapped in enigmas. They talked about urea, creatinine, uric acid, amino acids, polypeptides, indoles, phenoles, sulfates, hormones, phosphates, minerals, etc., as the causative agents. Among many other things, they even accused the deficiency of a certain chemicals, hormonal dysfunction and viral infection for uremia.

Tzi Kong Young, M.D., Ph.D. of the National Defense Medical Center, Taipei, Formosa, reported administration of saline solutions to induce diarrhea in 17 patients with uremia to remove uremic metabolites and to correct electrolyte derangements. Other scientists in this meeting also reported using charcoal, soil microbial enzymes, and various other compounds for use in the digestive tract in a bowel solute extraction technique (JAMA, 1978, vol. 231, no. 21, p. 2218) to relieve uremia. Drinking urine does not cause uremia, and the bowels function the same as the kidneys. Drinking urine causes a loose bowel movement within 30 to 45 minutes. It will clear and cleanse the entire bowel. At early stages of therapy, most of the urine consumed comes out through a rapid bowel movement. If one fasts totally, drinks plenty of water, practices urine massage, and drinks all of the urine that the kidneys produce, uremia will not develop. My own experience is proof of that.

We often see in nature that animals, especially dogs, cows, monkeys, goats, bulls, and deer, are constantly licking and drinking urine from their mates and other members of the herd. When they are thirsty, it is not uncommon to notice one animal drinking urine from another animal as it is passed. Animal physiologists have known for a long time that the camel and many desert animals produce very little urine. Most of the urea in urine gets recycled through the liver and converted into a new protein. It is possible that some of it may be converted into a protein or protein precursor. Urine itself contains many proteins and amino acids (see Chapter 7).

My Personal Experiments with AUT Show that It Is Safe If Proper Guidelines Are Followed and Combined with other hyperthermia and/or drugs

My own experiments on total autoimmune urine therapy, for one week, showed no raise in urea and related compounds (toxic metabolites) in the blood. I did not develop poisoning (uremia). My liver enzymes were normal. This shows that during autoimmune urine therapy (total or partial) there is no change in physiological functioning and values of the body. I have studied AUT for 25 years. I have examined all the scientific developments of the past and the present century. Based on my knowledge and experience, I firmly believe that autoimmune urine therapy does help to cure diseases and is not toxic if proper guidelines are followed. Autoimmune urine therapy has a place in medical pharmacology. It must be used under proper guidance, after the proper diagnosis is established. It is not a cure all therapy. I want to start experimentation with hyperthermia combined with AUT when I get the facilities. All my patients of poison ivy and many other skin condition got complete cure.

Use of AUT is not like some faith healer pitching a tent in the middle of nowhere, and healing people of all sorts of sickness and disappearing after collecting the money. Some of today's preachers claim that they can heal through the television. All one has to do is touch the television screen while they are preaching and send money. It is your belief that heals, not the faith healer (see Chapter 20 for more details).

After closely examining all the pros and cons, I am providing a scientific basis for the use of autoimmune urine therapy. I am including hyperthermia to enhance effects of urine therapy. I am not writing this book to put down any one group. The most important reason for writing this book is to take away the superstition surrounding autoimmune urine therapy. I will show a rational, scientific explanation of how and why autoimmune urine therapy works, how to use it, and where it has little value. I think AUT is a very useful method of treatment alone or in combination with hyperthermia with or without modern medical treatments (drugs, chemotherapy, radiation, surgery, hyperthermia, etc.)

Proponents and the opponents of AUT never gave any thought about using it as an adjunct therapy instead claims and disclaims. AUT has curative effects on many conditions on its own right without the help of other therapies. But combing other methods improves the odds of curtailing/curing the diseases. If other methods like hyperthermia and the drugs are not available, the AUT is one of the best choices of medical treatment available.

Opponents of Hyperthermia

It is interesting to note that the same type of skepticism has been raised about the efficacy of hyperthermia in curing various diseases. I talked to an expert in hyperthermia who uses it to treat cancers from Wisconsin on long distance call in June of 1990. He categorically and emphatically stated that the hyperthermia has no role in curing or curtailing AIDS. Same type of skepticism is expressed by majority of the scientists and the physicians I talked. I think they are judging the therapy prematurely and without putting into testing. If they follow the method I describe in this book they will be surprised at the outcome of the treatment. Hyperthermia itself will cure many diseases. If it is combined with AUT and drugs, the results will be very positive.

CHAPTER 7

WHAT IS URINE?

What does it Contain to Have Such Broad Healing Power?

He who masters two sciences of the pulse and the urine will possess almost all that is necessary for diagnosis and prognosis. Conversely, he who knows only one of these two sciences will be prone to a thousand errors, for in the study of diseases, the science of urine is as valuable as that of pulse.

Johannes Actuaries

The human body is a chemical, pharmaceutical, therapeutic and waste disposal factory. The kidneys are constantly absorbing, digesting, distilling, manufacturing, excreting, metabolizing, secreting, and assimilating thousands of compounds containing protein, carbohydrate, fats, metals, hormones, enzymes, organic, and inorganic compounds, and electrolytes. Many of these compounds and their byproducts are finally brought out through the kidneys in the form of urine. What do the kidneys do? They put out the end products of this human pharmaceutical factory and the end products of the body metabolism. They maintain a proper balance of the constituents of the body.

Mechanism of Urine Production (See Fig.3,4)

There are two kidneys in the body. They contain 2.5 million individual urine production units called nephrons (Fig.4). Each unit is capable of forming urine by itself. We can survive with one kidney. The diagram shows the functional unit (nephron) of the factory. The kidney receive 20% of the blood put out by the heart with each heart beat (Fig.4). A normal human body weighing 70 kg (154 pounds) produces 1400 ml (46 ounces) of urine a day. The heart pumps out 5600 ml of blood per minute, out of which 1200 ml of it pass through the kidneys each minute. Out of this 1200 ml of blood, 1 ml of urine is produced by the kidneys. The kidney puts out about 60 ml (2 ounces) of urine per hour. As the blood passes through the kidney filter (glomerulus), most of the constituents of blood pass through, except cells and most proteins. The liquid produced is called filtrate. It contains metabolites, excretions, secretions, hormones, parts of dead cell, (tumor cells and their products), parts or the whole of bacteria and virus (if there is infection), etc.

Each day 180 liters (396 pounds or 16 gallons) of filtrate (i.e., 125 ml/minute) is formed (twice the weight of the body). More than 90% of this filtrate is reabsorbed by the kidney tubules. The rest is passed as urine which is concentrated from 16 gallons of kidney filtrate from the blood. Substances with a molecular weight of 5200 will pass through the kidney as easily as any other substance dissolved in the blood plasma. Albumin, with a molecular weight of 69,000, does not pass except in disease states. It is impermeable to plasma proteins and cells in the blood, and is permeable to other dissolved substances in the blood. The kidney (glomerular) filtrate contains all the elements of blood, except the cellular contents. Only 0.03% (1/200th) of serum proteins pass into this filtrate.

Human Body: A 10 Gallon Tank with 75 Trillion Cells Floating in It

The human body contains 40 liters (10 gallons) of water. About 25 liters (6 gallons) are within the 75 trillion cells (intracellular fluid) that make up our body and its organs. The remaining 15 liters (4 gallons) surrounds the cells and is called extra cellular fluid. The 75 trillion cells of our body literally float in this 4 gallons of fluid outside the cells. Water makes up 57% of the body weight in adults and 75% in children. This extra-cellular fluid picks up all metabolites of the cells, their secretions and excretions. These enter the blood and pass through the kidney and come out selectively concentrated as urine. The fluid outside the cells is constantly exchanging various products (nutrients, hormones, enzymes, metabolic products, vitamins, oxygen, carbon dioxide, etc.) with the fluid inside the cell. All these products enter the blood circulation and are brought to the kidneys to be filtered out as urine. With hyperthermia and vigorous exercise, more of these substances enter the blood and come out in the urine. The urine is loaded with the healing and building substances. That is why it is important to practice AUT after exercise and hyperthermia.

Blood and Its Role in Urine Production

Of the five liters of blood in the body, two liters are red cells and the remaining three liters circulate as plasma. Every minute the entire volume of blood in the body passes through the heart to various tissues of the body and back to the heart. Blood is in constant motion like an eternal spring. The human blood circulates in a closed system of blood vessels and the heart. The contents of the blood, such as the white blood cells, plasma, oxygen, carbon dioxide, nutrients, electrolytes, enzymes, hormones, etc., are constantly moving in and out the blood vessels.

The plasma carries the nutrients to all the cells, picks up various cell secretions (hormones), and distributes them to all cells in our body. It brings the white blood cells and their products of the immune defense system (fighting soldiers) close to the site of the foreign material (antigen) or injuries. Without blood and lymph circulation, this function could not be done. Lymph vessels pick up proteins and other substances from the extracellular fluid and pour it back into blood circulation. This transfer and transportation is enhanced during hyperthermia and exercise. If we did not have blood and lymph vessels in our body to transport products of the immune system, it would be like an army without any means of transportation to reach and fight an aggressor.

Volume of Urine Produced

The volume of blood is very seldom altered, even in states of extreme dehydration or over hydration. The kidneys, along with sweat glands, play an important role in maintaining a steady blood volume. For example, when a large amount of water is ingested, it enters into the blood and is discarded as dilute urine. When less water is ingested or if water is lost by sweating, less urine is produced. This action by the kidneys preserves the volume of blood at a constant volume of 5000 ml.

The body of an average person under optimal physiological conditions puts out about 1 ml of urine every minute, amounting to about 1440 ml a day (roughly 1-1/2 liters, 15 to 21 ml's. per kilogram body weight). This can range anywhere from 600 ml to 2400 ml in 24 hours. If 24 hour urine output exceeds 2400 ml (80 ounces), physicians suspect kidney diseases such as diabetes mellitus, diabetes insipidus, nephritis, etc. Drinking large amounts of water, coffee, tea, or alcohol results in greater urine production. Tea and coffee contain chemicals (xanthine) which enhance urine output (diuretics).

Alcohol suppresses an antidiuretic hormone (ADH) produced in the brain, resulting in less absorption of filtrate in the kidney. This results in abundant urine formation. This hormone, under normal conditions, enhances the absorption of urine from the kidneys. Children produce three to four times as much urine as an adult. Under mild and moderate hyperthermia using jacuzzi, I found the urine production was reduced. If I had caffeinated or alcoholic beverages before entering the hot jacuzzi, the volume of urine produced was increased but still below what is expected under normal conditions. Don't be surprised if you pass copious amounts of urine 1-2 hours after hyperthermia if proper fluid balance is maintained.

Specific Gravity (SG)

The specific gravity of urine is between 1008 to 1035. It indicates the amount of solids in the urine, such as salts, sugar, proteins, etc. When the specific gravity becomes fixed at 1010, which is the same SG as plasma, kidneys have lost their ability to concentrate or dilute urine. They are not responding to physiological changes in the body. The SG of the urine increases with mild to moderate hyperthermia. With severe hyperthermia, with abundant fluid administration, the SG drops.

pH Of Urine (Is Urine Acid or Alkaline?)

Acidity or alkalinity or neutrality is represented as pH. A pH of 7 is neutral. Any value below a pH of 7 is acid. Any value above a pH of 7 is alkaline. For example, gastric juice is highly acid with a pH of 0.5 to 2.5. Normally, urine is acidic, with a pH of 4.5 to 6. The pH of urine varies between 4.5 and 9, meaning mildly acidic to highly alkaline. A high meat diet and some acidifying drugs such as ammonium chloride produce acid urine. The pH of the urine reflects the pH of the plasma (blood).

Alkaline urine (pH greater than 7) is rare. It is seen in people who eat large amounts of fruits and vegetables and very little meat protein. Ammonia splitting bacteria can also convert urine from acid to alkaline. One can test the pH of urine by using litmus paper commonly available in drug stores. If fresh urine is alkaline, barring high fruit and vegetable intake or drug use, it suggests kidney infection. If urine is allowed to sit for a long time before being tested, it becomes alkaline due to bacterial conversion. During and after hyperthermia the urine remains acidic.

Proteins In Urine

Substances in the plasma with a molecular weight of 5200 pass easily through the kidney. Other contents of plasma, such as albumin, globulin, glycoproteins from the lining of the genitourinary tract, mucoproteins, etc., pass through in renal disease states such as glomerulonephritis, nephrotic syndrome, toxemia of pregnancy, congestive heart failure, fever, anemia, liver disease, leukemia, various heart abnormalities, bone cancers, long periods of standing or walking, and strenuous exercise, etc. Urine contains abundant amounts of protein in one type of bone cancer (multiple myelomas) called Bence Jones protein. This protein precipitates when urine is heated to 50°C and redissolves when urine reaches the boiling point. This example shows that the kidney will allow many molecules having 69000 molecular weight or higher to pass through in various disease states. Therefore, disease-carrying organisms, their broken down parts, parts of dead body cells and their contents, secretions of various organs, hormones, etc., easily pass through the kidney. More of these substances and products are found in the urine during and after hyperthermia and exercise. This is an important point to remember when we consider why urine and hyperthermia works in curing many diseases.

Other Metabolic Substances In Urine

Urine contains many other metabolic substances. When these substances reach a high level in the blood plasma, they are excreted in urine. Some examples are the formation and the excretion of ketone bodies in diabetes and starvation, the production of bilirubin in jaundice (obstructive or hepatocellular jaundice), and the release of urobilinogen which occurs when there is a rapid destruction of red blood cells. Homogentisic acid is formed in alkaptonuria. The amino acid cystine, lysine, arginine and ornithine are found in cystinuria and in other renal disease, such as Fanconi's syndrome. Porphyrins are found in pernicious anemia, congenital porphyria, lead poisoning, etc. Many times, urine also contains unusual amounts of reducing sugars. This condition is called glycosuria (glucosuria, pentosuria, lactosuria, galactosuria, fructosuria). Eating large amounts of avocado results in urine containing d-Monoheptulose (a 7-carbon sugar). Contents of urine change during and after hyperthermia.

Kidney Hormones

The kidneys secrete many hormones. Hemopoietic factors hormone helps in red blood cells production. When the kidneys completely fail to function, the patient develops anemia. This hemopoietic factor is marketed now to treat anemia. The kidneys secrete an enzyme called urokinase. Urokinase helps dissolve blood clots in the blood vessels. Now it is used to dissolve the blood clots in the coronary arteries of the heart after a heart attack.

The kidneys secret another enzyme called renin (in the juxtaglomerular apparatus). Renin splits angiotensin-I from angiotensinogen, a serum globulin formed by the liver. This angiotensin-I is converted into angiotensin-II by serum angiotensinase. Angiotensin-II stimulates the adrenal glands to release a hormone called aldosterone. Release of aldosterone results in the retention of sodium in the blood. Extra sodium holds more water back in the blood, thereby elevating blood pressure. Thus renin plays an important role in control of arterial blood pressure. Whenever blood pressure drops, the kidneys produce more renin to bring the blood pressure back to normal. Angiotensinogen-II is destroyed in all body tissues, but in largest quantities in the kidneys and small intestine.

The kidneys produces other hormone-like substances called prostaglandins. Along with renin, it is involved in the regulation of salt and volume balance and blood pressure.

Hundreds of hormones produced by various endocrine glands and organs come out in the urine in various biologically degraded and undegraded forms (see the table at the end of the chapter). There are thousands of undefined molecules of various organic, inorganic chemicals, and body cell parts which come out of urine. Every year new compounds are discovered in the urine. Therefore, all I can say is that urine is not a foul smelling excreta but a "**living water with life.**"

Protein Metabolism and Urea Formation

The most important solute in urine is urea. About 20-30 grams of urea is formed in 24-hours and is proportional to protein intake. To understand urea formation, one needs to know something about the body proteins and their metabolism. The end product of protein digestion is amino acids. Amino acids are absorbed from the intestines and circulate as such in the blood (65 mg/100 cc plasma). Amino acids are the building blocks of the body and are transported into the cells through the cell membrane (by active transport or by facilitated diffusion). They are used in the cell to synthesize proteins used for various cell functions and stored as proteins. Once the cells are filled with a given protein, the DNA-RNA feed back control of the cells blocks further protein synthesis. Any additional amino acids in the body fluids are degraded and used for energy or stored as fat. Proteins come in and out of the cells as needed. When needed, with the help of lysosomal digestive enzymes in the cells, they are decomposed into amino acids and transported to the blood as amino acids.

The kidney, liver, and gut are the big reservoirs of the proteins. Growth hormone from the pituitary gland under the brain and insulin from the pancreas increase the formation of tissue protein, whereas the glucocorticoid hormone from the adrenal glands increases the circulating amino acids. When the tissues are depleted of proteins, plasma proteins can act as a source of rapid replacement of these proteins. Most plasma proteins are stored in the liver cells and macrophages. They can be split into amino acids and transported back into the blood to be utilized by cells.

It is important to remember that the formation of cellular proteins is the basis of life itself. Most of the proteins in a cell are in the form of enzymes which catalyze different chemical reactions in the cell. The genes (DNA) control the cell function. The DNA-controlled RNA literally produces hundreds of enzymes, hormones, proteins, and secretions. Degradation of the amino acids takes place in the liver where they are used as energy or stored as fat in the process called deamination. In the liver two molecules of ammonia are released during deamination. They combine with one molecule of carbon dioxide to form urea (2NH3 + CO2 = H2N - C - NH2 (urea) + H20). In the absence of liver function, the ammonia accumulates in the blood. It is extremely toxic to the brain, resulting in hepatic coma and death.

All the urea in the human body is essentially synthesized in the liver. The urea diffuses from the liver to the blood and body fluids, and is excreted in urine. Eighteen of the 20 deaminated amino acids can be used by the cell for energy (ATP production) to support various activities, or it can be converted into glucose or glycogen (gluconeogenesis). Nineteen of the 20 amino acids can be converted to keto acids and then fat (ketogenesis). Only about 40% of the urea in the urine is absorbed back into circulation from the kidneys as well as from the intestines when it is ingested. Creatinine is not absorbed. About 86% of urate ions are reabsorbed. Sulfates, phosphates, and nitrates behave the same way as urate ions.

Effect of Starvation on the Proteins in the Body

When a person does not eat any protein, up to 20-30 grams of body protein is degraded to amino acid, deaminated and oxidized every day (obligatory loss). Therefore, to prevent loss of protein from the body, one should eat at least 20-30 grams each day. To be on the safe side 60-75 grams are recommended. Except for this loss during starvation, the body uses carbohydrates and fats for energy as long as they are available. That is why carbohydrates and fats are called protein sparers. As the body loses fats and carbohydrates, it starts using proteins rapidly, up to 125 grams a day instead of the usual 20 - 30 grams for energy needs. When the body loses more than 50% of its proteins from muscles, bones, brain, and other cells of various organs, death usually follows. During hyperthermia, use of carbohydrates, fats, and proteins is increased many folds. But drinking urine will reduce the protein loss. People can sustain life with urine and water for 100 days or more.

Color and Smell of Urine

The color of urine depends on the pH, concentration, pigments, diseases, length of time the urine is exposed to the air, food habits and the medications taken. Malingerers color their urine by adding blood, colored crepe paper and dyes, or by eating colored foods. The normal color of the urine is pale yellow to deep gold (amber). The principle pigments (coloring agents) of urine are urochrome, (made up of urobilin), urobilinogen, and a peptide of unknown structure. The other pigments which give the urine this color are uroerythrin (derived from melanin pigments from the skin), uroporphyrin, and riboflavin (vitamin).

The smell of urine depends on the food eaten, medicines taken, and the diseases suffered. The urine usually smells ammoniacal. All of us are aware of the smell of asparagus after eating it. Ammonia in the urine is manufactured in the kidney from the glutamine and an amino acid from the blood. If the urine is alkaline, formation and output of ammonia in the urine is reduced.

The table at the end of the chapter gives the usual urine coloration under various conditions (*Hospital Physician*, no. 3, 1978, p. 22)

Urine during Hyperthermia

Contents and color of urine varies depending on the metabolic state, heart functioning, water levels of the body. For example, during hyperthermia, with proper fluid balance, the amount of urine produced is increased. Further it contains more components of dead cells microbes, lymphokines, enzymes, hormones, immunoglobulins, electrolytes etc. It contains less metabolic products and urea if proper fluid balance is maintained. That is why the urine during and after hyperthermia is a rich source of antigen. It will stimulate the immune system immensely to fight diseases. During mild and moderate hyperthermia, without intravenous fluid administration, results in less amount of concentrated urine production. The same effect is seen after exercise. During hyperthermia or exercise, a lot of fluid is lost in the sweat. The blood circulating in the kidney is reduced and the circulation is increased 3-5 times.

Color of the Urine under Various Normal Abnormal Conditions

Urine Color	Conditions
1.Colorless	Drinking too much water (over hydration), Diabetes Mellitus, Diabetes Insipidus
2.Deep orange	Drinking less or no water, Dehydration by sweating/diarrhea/severe exercise
3.Milky color	Pus in the urine (pyuria) Lymph in the urine (chyluria)
4.Red color	Broken red cells in urine hemoglobinuria), Massive destruction of muscles (myoglobinuria), Long standing mercury & lead poisoning, Intact red blood cells in urine (hematuria) Beets or blackberries due to anthocyanin pigment
5.Reddish brown	Urobilinogen in high quantity, porphyrins (porphyria), Rhubarb, aloe (seaweed) and flava beans
6.Brown	Argyrol, Nitrofurantoin, Primaquine, Chloroquine, Furazolidone, Metronidazole
7.Blue to blue green to green	Jaundice Urinary derivative of tryptophan,indole, Amitriptyline, Anthraquinolin, Arbutin, flavin derivatives, Indigo blue, Tetralin, Thymol, Phenol, Maol, methylene blue, resorcinol, salol, toluidine blue
8.Black	Due to presence of homogentisic acid (a product of protein phenylalanine and tyrosine metabolism - called alcaptonuria) b-hydroxyphenylpyruvic acid (Tyrosinosis)

Color of Urine under Various Normal and Abnormal Conditions

Urine Color	Condition
9.Brownish Black	Melanin pigment (from skin), Acidification of haemoglobin pigment derived from red blood cells
10.Yellow	Methyldopa (Aldomet) Cascara, Pyrogallol, iron, sorbitol,Methocarbonal(Robaxin),Sena, Phenylhydrazine
11.Orange	By drugs such as phenacetin, quinacrine, Riboflavin Obstructive jaundice, Eating food containing yellow turmeric as seen in East India, Normal color of urine (light yellow), Santonin given for round worms and hook worm infestation of intestines, Salicylazosulfapyridine (azulfidine), Phenazopyridine (pyridium), Azogantrisin, Azogantonol, Ethoxazene (serenium)
12.Pale blue green(rainbow urine)	Dewitts pills made by international corporation, over the counter drug recommended for backache, aches all over the body, urinary tract infection. It contains about six different compounds of questionable value (Salicylamide, Pot. nitrate, uva ursi, Bachu leaves extract, caffeine, methylene blue)
13."Cloudy" on standing	Indicates urates are precipitated in acid urine and phosphates in alkaline urine
14.Orange to yellow to dark greenish brown	Indicates oxidation of urobilinogen pigment in the urine by exposure to on standing in air

Physiological Values of Urine and Its Contents

Urine is an end-product of kidney function. A single specimen, or even a timed collection often cannot provide enough information about the dynamics of kidney function. Several test procedures are available to investigate the kidney filtration unit (glomerular) flow rate and tubular excretory capacity. The following table gives the normal physiological values of a 24-hour urine collection.

1. Addis count

   WBC 1,800,000; RBC 5000,000; casts (hyaline) 0-5000
   (Rinse bottle with 10% neutral formalin and discard excess 12 hr specimen.)

2. Albumin

   Qualitative - Negative
   (Single specimen)

   Quantitative - 10-100 mg/24 hr
   (24 hr specimen)

3. Aldosterone

   2-23 μg/24 hr
   (24-hr specimen; keep refrigerated)

4. Amino acid nitrogen

   100-290 mg/24 hr
   (24 hr specimen; collect in thymol; refrigerate)

5. Ammonia

   700 mg/24 hr 4 to 75 mEq/L) (0.4 to 1.0 g 24 hr)
   (24 hr specimen)

6. Amylase

   2-50 Wohlgemuth u/ml
   (Single specimen)

7. Amylase, total in 24 hr
   6-30 Wohlgemuth u/ml
   Up to 5000 Somogyi u/24 hr
   (24 hr specimen)

8. Bence-Jones protein
   Negative
   (First morning specimen)

9. Bilirubin
   Negative
   (Single specimen)

10. Blood, occult
    Negative
    (Single specimen)

11. Calcium
    2.5 to 7.5 mEq/L
    0.1 to 3.0 gm/24 hr
    Sulkowitch: Positive 1+
    (Single specimen)

    Quantitative: 30-150 mg/24 hr (average diet)
    100-250 mg/24 hr (high-calcium diet)
    (24 hr specimen)

12. Catecholamine
    Less than 230 μg in 24 hr
    (24 hr specimen; use 1 ml concentrated H2SO4 as preservative)

13. Chloride
    110-250 mEq/24 hr
    (24 hr specimen)

14. Coproporphyrin
 50-200 μg/24 hr
 Children: 0-80 μg/24 hr
 (24 hr specimen in 5 Gm of Na2HCO3)

15. Creatine
 0.3 to 0.8 gm/24 hr
 Less than 200 mg in 24 hr, or less than 6% of creatinine
 Pregnancy: up to 12 % of creatinine
 Children under 1 yr: may equal creatinine
 Children over 1 yr: up to 30% of creatinine
 (24 hr specimen)

16. Creatinine
 Females : 0.8-1.7 Gm/24 hr
 Males : 1-1.9 Gm/24 hr
 (24 hr specimen)

17. Estrogens
 Females : 4-60 μg/24 hr
 Males : 4-25 μg/24 hr
 (24 hr specimen; refrigerate)

18. Fishberg concentration test
 Specific gravity: 1.022 to 1.032
 (Collect specimens at 7, 8 and 10 a.m.)

19. Fishberg dilution test
 Volume of 40 ml in first hour with specific gravity 1.001 to 1.003 (Collect 4 hourly specimens after drinking 1200 ml of water)

20. Glucose
Qualitative: Negative
(Single specimen)
Quantitative: Less than 100 mg/1000 ml
(24 hr specimen)
Hippuric acid: 0.04 to 0.05 gm/24 hr

21. Gonadotrophic hormone, pituitary
10 to 15 mouse uterine u/24 hr
(24 hr specimen; collect with toluene)

22. H+: (hydrogen ions)
4 x 10 to power of 8 or 4 x 10 to power of 6 mEq/L

23. 17-Hydroxycortico-steriods
Females: 2-8 mg/24 hr
Males: 3-20 mg/24 hr
(24 hr specimen tranquilizers interfere)

24. 5-Hydroxyindoleacetic acid
2-9 mg/24 hr
(24 hr specimen; tranquilizers interfere)

25. Iron
0.2 mg/24 hr

26. 17-Ketosteriods
24-hr excretion:
Females: age 10, 1-4 mg; age 20-30, 4-16 mg; age 50, 3-9 mg;
age 70, 1-7 mg
Males: age 10, 1-4 mg; age 20-30, 6-26 mg; age 50, 5-18 mg;
age 70, 2-10 mg

27. Lead
0.021-0.038 mg/L
24 hr specimen

28. Magnesium
    0.1-2.00 g
    (acid to alkaline)

29. pH
    4.8 to 7.8
    (Single specimen)

30. Phenylpyruvic acid
    Negative
    (Single specimen)

31. Peptides
    0.3 to 0.7 gm/24 hr

32. Phosphates
    0.9-1.6 Gm/24 hr (20-50 mEq/L)
    (24 hr specimen)

33. Porphobilinogen
    Negative
    (Single specimen)

34. Potassium
    25-100 mEq/24 hr (1.5 to 2.0 Gm
    (24 hr specimen)

35. Pregnanediol
    Children: negative; Females - 1-8 mg/24hr;
    Males: 0-1 mg/24 hr
    (24 hr specimen; refrigerate)

36. Pregnanetriol
    Children: Less than 0.5 mg/ 24 hr.
    Females: 0.5-2 mg/24 hr.
    Males - 1.0-2.0 mg/24 hr
    (24 hr specimen; refrigerate)

37. Protein
Bence Jones protein: Negative
(First morning specimen)
Qualitative: Negative
(Single specimen)
Quantitative: 10-100 mg/24 hr
(24 hr specimen)

38. Serotonin
See 5-Hydroxyindoleacetic acid

39. Sodium
About 110 mEq/24 hr (2 to 4 Gm)
(24 hr specimen)

40. Specific gravity
1.002-1.030
(Single specimen)
1.015-1.025
(24 hr specimen)

41. Sulfate-Organic
0.06 to 0.2 Gm/24 hr

42. Sulfate-inorganic
0.6 to 1.8 Gm/24 hr

43. Sugars
Negative
(Single specimen)

44. Urea clearance
Maximum : 75 ml
Standard: 54 ml
(Serum and urine)

45. Urea
6-18-30 Gm/24 hrs

46. Uric acid
0.5-2.00 Gm/24 hr
(24 hr specimen)

47. Urobilinogen
Semiquantitative: Up to 1 Ehrlich u/2 hr
(2 hr specimen; collect between 1 & 3 p.m.)

Quantitative: 1.0-4.0 mg/24 hr
(24 hr specimen; collect in dark container with 5 Gm of Na2HCO3)

48. Vanilmandelic acid
0.7-6.8 mg/24 hr
(24 hr specimen in 3 ml 24% H2SO4; omit fruit and coffee 2 days before test)

49. Indican:
4-20 mg 4 hr
(24 hr specimen)

50. Volume
Adults: 1000-1500 ml/24 hr
(about 15-21 ml/kg body wt)
Children: 3 to 40 times a much as adults
per kg of body wt

The following tables gives various contents of urine so far identified. It is obvious from these tables that the urine contains hundreds of organic and inorganic compounds. No wonder urine has such a life sustaining and disease curing qualities.

During hyperthermia, the contents of urine will be different. The concentrations of various components of urine also varies hours and days after moderate to severe hyperthermia. The microbes and disease afflicted cells killed by hyperthermia are gradually removed from the tissue spaces and moved to the blood and lymph vessels. These substances are excreted through the urine gradually. That is why I strongly recommend total AUT during and many days after hyperthermia.

Normal Adult Urine Values in mg in 24 hour urine an balanced diet (Modified from Geigy Documenta Scientific Tables, 6th ed. 1962)
g=grams, mg=milligrams, μg=micrograms, L=liter, dl=deciliter

Data	Mean	Range
Dry wight	-	55-70g
Proteins	-	
Total proteins		20-100
Mucoproteins		
Men	146	99-193
Women	106	66-146
Glycoproteins	-	1-11mg/100ml
Nitrogen		
Total nitrogen	15g	10-20g
Ammonia-N	-	0.4-1g
Amino acid-N,total	349	267-431
Amino acids		
Alanine	27μg/ml	-
ß Aminoisobutyric acid	7μg/ml	-
Arginine		
Total:Men	47	37-57
Women	33	17-50
Free: Men	24	.4-48
Women	17	6-29
Serine		
Total	-	0.35-1.4mg/kg
Free	-	0.21-0.52mg/kg
Taurine	156	-
Threonine		
Total:Men	83	42-125
Women	64	27-102
Free: Men	60	28-92
Women	52	10-94
Cystine (free)	88	38-138

Data	Mean	Range
Organic bases		
Creatinine		
Adults		1.0-3.0 g
Old people: Men	2g	0.26-0.69 g
Women	0.48g	0.035-1.0g
Ethanolamine	0.46g	-
Guanidine	3μg/ml	10-20
	-	
Tryptophan(amino acids)		
Total: Men	23	13-33
Women	17	8-25
Free: Men	21	10-32
Women	16	5-27
Tyrosine		
Total: Men	56	38-73
Women	41	19-64
Free: Men	44	32-57
Women	33	19-47
Valine		
Total: Men	30	16-45
Women	28	13-43
Free: Men	20	8-33
Women	17	6-28
Organic bases		
Allantoin	-	25-30
Choline	-	6-9

Data	Mean	Range
Enzymes		
Amylase	3095units	1047-5143units
Uropepsin	415	98-835
Inorganic constituents		
Chloride		
Phosphorus	7368	-
Sulfur (as SO3)	1100	-
Total		
Inorganic	-	2000-3400
Organic(neutral)	-	1700-2700
Alkylsulfuric acids	-	200-400
Calcium	-	150-300
Potassium	-	141-365
Magnesium	2740	-
Sodium	103	33-307
	4615	-
Aluminum	78μg/L	14-142μg/L
Lead	27μg/L	0-55μg/L
Iron	0.045	-
Iodine	-	0.018-0.483
Copper		
Adults	0.018	0.0035-0.0325
Children	0.048	0.0154-0.0806
Manganese	10μg/L	-
Nickel	0.1mg/L	-
Silver	-	trace
Tin	11μg/L	0-31μg/L
Zinc	0.457	-
Cells		
Bacteria		present
Hyaline Casts		0-5000
WBC		1,800,000
Erythrocytes		500,000

Data	Mean	Range
Glutamine(amino acids)	32μg/ml	-
Glutamic acid		
Total: Men	250	15-484
Women	249	45-452
Free: Men	235	108-363
Women	202	56-348
Glycine		
Total	405	139-671
Free	226	131-321
Histidine		
Total:Men	284	69-499
Women	170	57-283
Free: Men	256	82-429
Women	162	38-287
Hydroxyproline		
Total	23	-
Free	0.55	-
Isoleucine		
Total:Men	11	7-16
Women	12	4-19
Free: Men	8	3-13
Women	6	2-11
Aspartic acid		
Total:Men	113	16-210
Women	92	30-153
Free: Men	75	0-155
Women	54	21-87

Data	Mean	Range
Leucine(amino acids)		
Total: Men	28	12-44
Women	22	11-33
Free: Men	30	6-34
Women	13	4-22
Lysine		
Total: Men	102	44-160
Women	97	29-165
Free: Men	57	15-100
Women	57	7-108
Methionine		
Total: Men	7	4-9
Women	6	2-9
Free: Men	4	1-7
Women	3	0.6-5.0
Phenylalanine		
Total: Men	29	13-44
Women	24	11-37
Free: Men	19	13-24
Women	15	4-26
Proline		
Total: Men	43	24-62
Women	50	20-79
Free: Men	35	19-52
Women	33	6-60

Data	Mean	Range
Carbohydrates and related substances		
Sugars	-	500-1500
Glucose	72	16-132
Pentoses		
Ribulose	1mg/L	-
Xylulose	4mg/L	-
Inositol		
Total	-	35-85mg/L
Myoinositol	-	22-30mg/L
Scyllitol	-	15-22mg/L
Glucuronic acid(Total)		
Men	6	5-7
Women	4	3-4
Boys	6	7-8
Girls	6	5-7
Amino sugars	84	60-108
Lipids		
Free fatty acids	-	8-50
Cholesterol	-	20-140μg/dl
Complete urine		
Urine without sediment	-	20-90μg/dl
Intermediary metabolites		
Acetone bodies	19	14-24
Citric acid	678	128-1228
Homogentisic acid	0	-
Lactic acid	-	100-600
Oxalic acid	-	20-40
Phenols	437	260-636
Pyruvic acid	100	-
Succinic acid	-	2-11

Data	Mean	Range
Blood pigments & other pigments		
Hemoglobin	0	-
Methemoglobin	0	-
Myohemoglobin	0	-
Porphyrins	-	-
Aminolevulic acid	3mg/L	0.1-6mg/L
Porphobilinogen	1mg/L	0.0-2mg/L
Coproporphyrin	0.07mg/L	0-0.15mg/L
Uroporphyins	-	0-15μg/L
Urobilinogen	-	0-4
Bilirubin	5	-
Guanidinoacetic acid	30	-
Hippuric acid	0.7g	0.1-1.0g
Imidazoles:		
low-protein diet(40g)	286	150-300
high-protein diet(110g)	443	320-600
Indican;3-ind.H2SO4.	-	5-10
Kynurenine		
20 yrs	0.096/dl	0.014-0.178/dl
47 yrs	0.207/dl	0.017-0.431/dl
Purine bases	-	10-60
Urea	-	20-35g
Uric acid	528	80-976

Show me a medicine or pharmaceutical product which contains all the above products in physiological proportions and many more hundreds of unidentified products. Even if we spend a billion dollars, this product cannot be manufactured. Every year new product are identified in the urine. That is why urine has healing qualities and along with water sustains life without any adverse effects. Urine is totally non allergic. **That is why I call it the Living Water with Life** and it is even free.

FIGURE 3: SHOWS THE KIDNEYS (URINE PRODUCING), URETERS (URINE DRAINING), BLADDER (URINE STORING) AND URETHRA (URINE EXITING) OF URINARY SYSTEM.

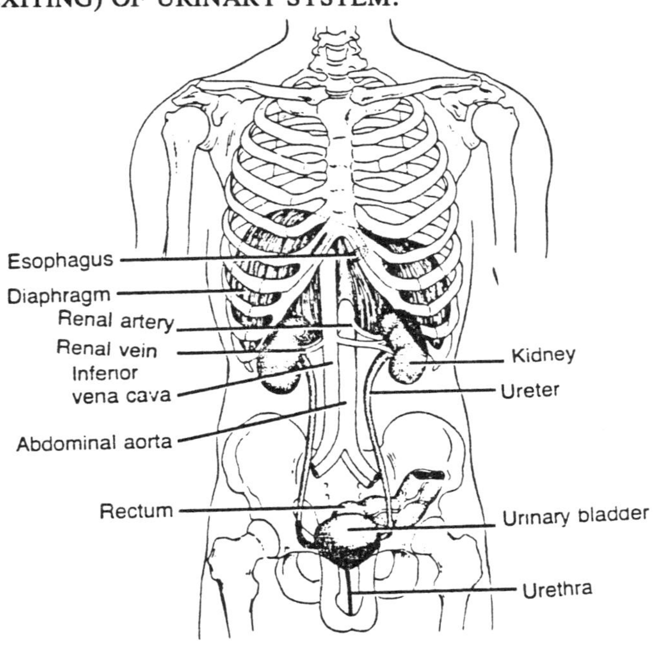

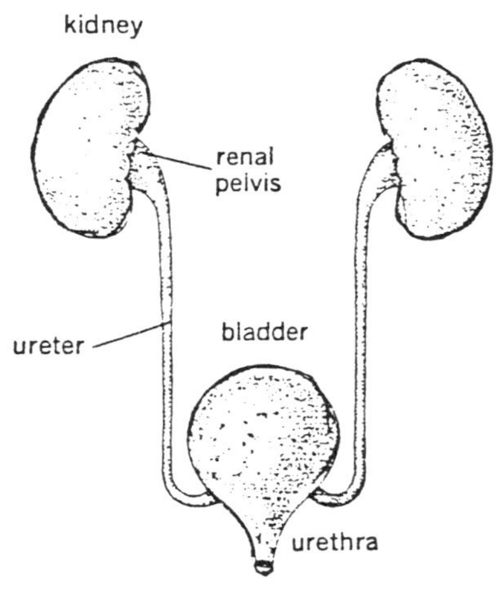

FIGURE 4: SHOWS THE INSIDE OF THE KIDNEY AND URINE PRODUCING UNIT (NEPHRON) OF THE KIDNEY.

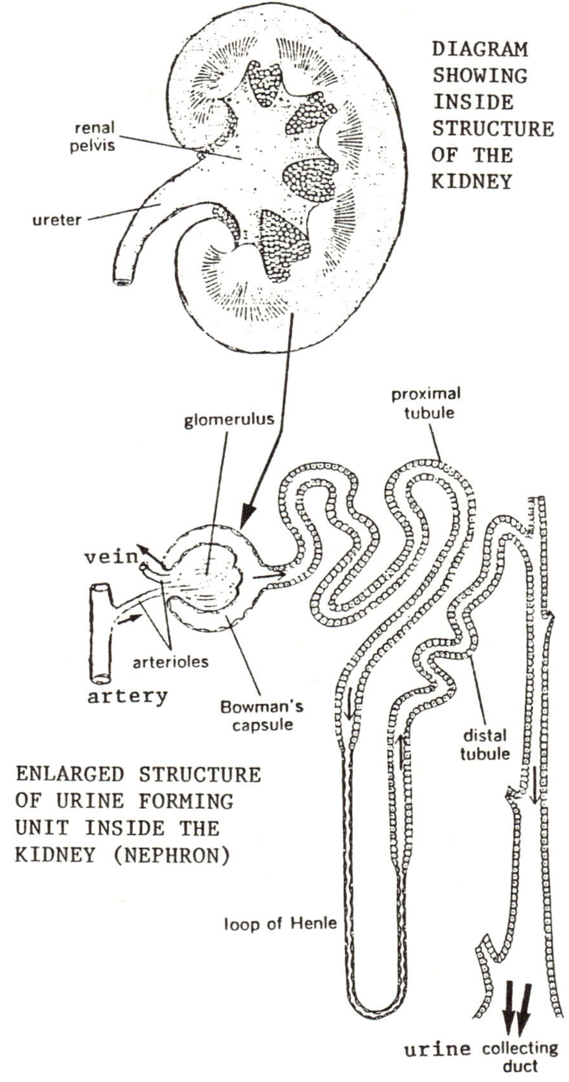

CHAPTER 8

BODY DEFENSE MECHANISM

Immune Defense System
How body fights diseases

Resist the devil and he will flee from you.
James 4:7

Immunity is only one of the weapons in the basic struggle for life and denotes the resistance which each organism offer against aggression by another.
William C. Boyd
Fundamentals of Immunology, 1947

This chapter describes various components of the immune system in our body, how it defends our body against the intruders, and how to help this system and enhance its activity by Auto Immune Urine (AUT) therapy and hyperthermia to cure or curtail a disease.

It was known for centuries that recovery from infectious illnesses resulted in the ability to resist reinfections. This phenomenon was observed before the discovery of the germ theory of infectious diseases. The Chinese physicians in the 11th Century, B.C. knew that the inhalation of smallpox crusts prevented later development of the disease. On June 26, 1821,the Boston physician Rabdice Boylston inoculated his son and two slaves by putting the small pox crust on the cut skin. He learned this method from a

Boston clergyman named Cotton. The clergyman learned this method of small pox prevention from an African slave. Many slaves underwent this procedure in Africa before they were traded. Small pox scab powder was introduced into the skin of women in the Middle East. This was done to prevent smallpox attacks and its devastating effect on beauty. This practice reached England in the 18th century.

In 1798 Edward Jenner, as medical student noted that the milk maids with cowpox were resistant to smallpox. He inoculated a young boy with the cowpox crusts which later protected the same boy from smallpox. Thus the modern era of immunization was born. It took almost another 100 years for Louis Pasteur to develop preventive immunization against rabies by using a killed or weakened virus. He named this preventive immunization material "vaccine" in honor of Jenner's contribution (vaccine from vacca which is latin for cow). These developments led to the modern scientific discipline called immunology. As a result many infectious diseases are eradicated, others controlled, and millions of human life saved.

To understand autoimmune urine therapy, it is important to know how the human body protects itself from various diseases. This protective system is called the immune defense system. I will describe this immune defense system and how it operates in health and disease. The description is quite technical and needs biology background to understand.

Evolution of the Immune System

Primitive animals developed a system by which degenerated portions of cells could be used to manufacture new cells. They picked up old, damaged cells and their fragments and digested them (phagocytosis), creating new growth in the cell (e.g. amoeba). As evolution advanced, these cells and their descendants developed similar functions. They would pick up foreign organisms and protein that had gained entrance into the body. This original phagocytic cell, the amebocyte, is like lymphocytes and macrophages of the immune system in our body. With further development, these cells evolved into the immune system. This system is very complex and contains many varieties of white blood cells, enzymes, secretions (lymphokines), and many organs.

Components of the Immune System (Fig.5)

The immune system in humans consists of:

1. Specific lymphoid organs (thymus gland, spleen).
2. Masses of lymphoid tissue embedded in various organs all over the body (lymph nodes).
3. Isolated lymphoid cells infiltrating the epithelial and connective tissues of the body.
4. White blood cells circulating in blood and lymph. These can be compared to a rapid mobile army traveling to the area of insult.

The lymphoid tissue (lymph nodes) plays an important role in the body immune defense mechanism. They are strategically located. For example, lymphoid tissue is located within the walls of the gut which comes in contact with antigens from the gut (from food and liquids). Lymphoid tissue in the throat (tongue, tonsils, and adenoids. See Fig. 5) interrupts antigens invading by the way of the respiratory tract and mouth (air and food). Lymph nodes located in the neck, armpit and groin interrupt the antigens (microbes etc) from the peripheral parts of the body through the skin and mucous membranes. The lymphoid tissue of the spleen, liver and bone marrow plays an important role in intercepting harmful antigenic agents circulating in the blood.

The cells of the immune system are strategically housed in blood, tissues, thymus gland, lymph nodes and the spleen (called internal secretory system). They are also located in the body tracts exposed to external environment such as respiratory, gastrointestinal, and genitourinary system (called the external secretory system). AUT and hyperthermia stimulates all the organ which house the immune system and enhances their activity.

Substances which Confront the Immune System (Antigens, Immunogens)

Most substances which encounter and activate our body's immune defense system arise from the outside world. Among the substances are a myriad of foreign substances ranging from simple low molecular weight chemicals to the most complex disease causing microbial agents. The immune system is also stimulated by substances within the body. Examples are: transplanted cells, viral or chemically altered cells, and cancer cells. Substances which evoke the immunologic response are called, immunogens or antigens. Some of these antigens are capable of producing a response without any help. Others many have to be attached to a protein (hapten) before an immune response is evoked (e.g. penicillin allergy).

Examples of environmental agents which act as antigens arousing an immune response are numerous. They include microbes (bacteria, virus, fungi, spirocheta, protozoa), plant products (tree, grass, pollen, poison ivy,), food products (eggs, milk, nuts, fish, cheese, chocolate), animal products (dander, blood, serum), insects (bee stings, spider bites, and other poisonous insect attacks), biological products (vaccines, blood products, transplanted organs, malignant cells), drugs (penicillin and a host of antibiotics), and chemicals (food additives, preservatives, dyes, metals, toxic substances).

Hyperthermia and Enhanced Antigen Output

Hyperthermia induction is one of the best way to induce high antigen output in the urine. When these are taken orally, enhances the output of antibodies. During hyperthermia, the antigens, immaterial of their source are partially denatured. This processes of denaturing enhances their effect as antigens and resulting in intense stimulation of antibodies. Hyperthermia enhances the liberation and circulation of antigens as described in chapter 1. Many of these antigens find their way into urine. The urine is loaded with the antigens. When they are taken orally, they are denatured by the digestive enzymes. They are absorbed by the digestive system, and presented to the immune defense cells. This results in intense stimulation of immune system which acts against the offending agent or microbe.

Antigens (immunogens) and Their Effect

Antigens are usually proteins or large polysaccharide (with a molecular weight of 800 or more). The effect of an antigen depends on its type and location. For example, antigen contact with the skin (target cells) produces dermatitis (poison ivy). Antigens specific to mucosal cells cause bleeding within the digestive tract. Antigens specific to smooth muscle cells cause diarrhea and vomiting. Antigen contact with glandular cells cause increased mucous production which results in tearing and the nasal dripping experienced in spring allergies. Antigens specific to the respiratory tract cause a cough due to mucus production and an asthma like attack due to bronchospasm. Their contact with the endothelial cells lining blood vessel causes increased intercellular spaces (pores) allowing more fluid to escape from the blood outside the vessel resulting in edema. Red blood cell contact result in their destruction resulting in anemia. These are examples of what happens when antigens comes in contact with the skin, digestive, respiratory, and circulatory system. There is hardly any organ in the body which is not targeted by one or more antigens.

How Antigens Stimulate Immune System to produce Antibodies

The mechanism by which antigens stimulate the immune system is not clearly known. One theory states that antigens serve as templates which furnish a model (i.e. instructions) for the manufacture of antibodies by competent immune cells (plasma cells). According to another theory, antigens act as instructive agents. They produce specific and inheritable changes in antibody producing cells. This results in clones or strains of cells. Their descendants are capable of producing specific antibodies when stimulated by that same specific antigen years later. These clones of cells and their antibodies fight the diseases in our body and are responsible for long term immunity. AUT and hyperthermia stimulates the division of clones of cells, production of antibodies thus enhances short and long term immunity.

Outlines of the Body Defense Against Intruders

During the course of the immune system evolution, several specific and nonspecific immunologic mechanisms appeared. They were placed throughout the body at strategic places, to protect the target cells. The important nonspecific response and the body's first line of defense is phagocytosis. This means ingestion of the antigen by macrophages, neutrophils, and eosinophils with a subsequent inflammatory response. These cells engulf, digest and eliminate the antigen. The way phagocytes destroy the eaten antigen is complex. Phagocytes contain more than a dozen enzymes. They act on the ingested antigens. This results in inactivation and dissolution of the foreign antigen. Many of these white cells die, resulting in pus formation. By attacking the antigen entering the target cells, these cells localize infections and prevent their spread to other parts of the body.

There are a second class of cells called mediator cells in our body. They release chemicals, such as histamines, serotonins, kinins, prostaglandins, thromboxanes, leukotrienes, chemotactic factors of anaphylaxis, slow reactive factor of anaphylaxis, platelet activating factors, and lysosomal enzymes. These mediator cells are mast cells (derived from hemopoietic stem cells), basophils, platelets, enterochromoffin cells, and neutrophils. When the antigen comes in contact with the mediator cells, they release many or all of the above mediator chemicals. These mediator chemicals act on target cells resulting in many adverse conditions such as allergy, anaphylaxis, asthma, diarrhea, etc. and act on phagocytic cells, increasing their movement to the site of the irritant (chemotaxis).

A third specific immune system with many different functions has also evolved in our body. It consists of the lymphoid system with lymphocytes. It produces specific antibodies to defend against specific antigens. These antibodies provide the long term immunity from the ravages of infections such as tetanus, smallpox, polio, typhoid, cholera, measles, etc. Failure of this system results in cancers. Acquired immunity which develops after vaccination or exposure to disease is the product of lymphoid tissue. When the lymphoid system fails, foreign environmental factors attack the human body. This results in disease and death. Failure of this specific immune system (lymphoid system) is responsible for almost 90,000 deaths (by 1990) in the U.S.A. due to AIDS. All of these immune mechanisms are needed for human survival and their activity can be enhanced by mild to moderate hyperthermia and AUT.

Different Cells of the Immune Defense System (Fig.6)

The cells participating in the immune defense system are called white blood cells (WBC). The human body contains millions of these white blood cells. The circulating blood contains red blood cells (which carry oxygen), white blood cells (body defense system), and platelets (plays major role in blood clotting). There are 7,000 white blood cells (WBC) in every cubic millimeter of blood. They are as follows:

1) Granulocytes:
   - Polymorphonuclear leukocytes 62%
   - Eosinophils 23%
   - Basophils 0.4%
2) Monocytes (becomes macrophages) 5.3%
3) Lymphocytes (80% T Type, 20% B Type) 30%

   Granulocytes contain small granules (pockets of lysosomal enzymes) within their cytoplasm.

Mother cells (pluripotential stem cells. Fig. 6), located in red bone marrow, produce red blood cells, platelet precursors, and myeloid stem cells. The latter differentiate into monocytes (macrophages), granulocytes (neutrophils, basophils, eosinophils, mast cells), and lymphoid stem cells. The lymphoid stem cells differentiate into B cell precursors, giving rise to memory B cells and plasma cells. And T cell precursors, give rise to T_4 helper/inducer cell and T_8 cytotoxic cell/suppressor cell.

Mast cells play an important role in allergies. They are located outside the circulating blood. The function of the macrophages and granulocytes is the first line of defense, i.e., phagocytosis (swallowing of the invading foreign antigens, virus, bacteria, dead cells, cancer cells, pollen, etc.). Lymphocytes are involved in the specific immune defense system and acquired immunity.

T and B Type Lymphocytes (Fig.6)

The lymphocyte precursor cells (stem cells) are derived from the yolk sac in the embryo and bone marrow in adults. One set of stem cells migrate to the thymus gland and differentiate to become T cells. Second set probably migrate to bone marrow (similar to bursa Fabricius) to become B cells. Here they undergo antigen independent proliferation, as T and B lymphocytes respectively. Both T and B lymphocytes re-enter the blood stream and populate lymph nodes, spleen and connective tissues of the body. When these specific T and B lymphocytes meet appropriate antigens they are stimulated to transform, proliferate, and differentiate. They give rise to activated T lymphocytes which provide cell mediated immunity; B lymphocytes and plasma cells which provide humoral (antibody) immunity.

As a result of antigen stimulation, lymphocytes carry the memory of the primary response. These cells have the capacity to mount an attack upon successive exposures to the same infection (antigen) at any time. Such an immunological surveillance is only possible because lymphocytes are able to move freely throughout the body. The effector lymphocyte and plasma cell precursors are seeded by blood and lymph throughout the immune system and connective tissues of the body. The plasma cell precursors are localized in large numbers in the intestines (lamina propria) where they develop into mature plasma cells. They are involved in the synthesis and release of antibodies against antigens.

Types T Lymphocytes and Their Function

The T lymphocytes are further divided into three sub groups based on their function:

1. Cytotoxic T cells or killer T cells (T_8 cells). The receptor protein on the surface of the cytotoxic cell causes them to bind tightly to cells which contain virus and bacteria, cancer cells, transplant cells. They swell and release cytotoxic (toxic to cells) substances (lysosomal enzymes) directly into the attacked cell there by killing them.
2. The second group is called Helper/inducer T cells (T_4 cells). They make up about 70% of the circulating T cells. These cells

have emerged as the prime participant in the immune defense. They increase the activation of B cells, cytotoxic T cells, and suppressor T cells. By secreting a substance called interlukin-II and alpha interferon, inducer T cells increase the activities of all the T cells including the helper cells and macrophages.

3. The third group is called suppressor and regulator T cells (T_8 cells). Not much is known about these cells. They are capable of suppressing the function of cytotoxic and helper T cells. Thus they keep them from causing an excessive immune reaction which can damage the body (immune tolerance).

Activation of T and B cells

There are millions of preformed B lymphocytes and T lymphocytes. They are capable of forming highly specific antibodies (humoral response by B cells) and T cells (cellular response) when activated by an appropriate antigen. They are like molds, producing an exact replica capable of performing that particular function. Only the specific antigen with which it can react will activate them. For example, if a B lymphocyte is stimulated by a specific antigen, the dormant clones of B cells will enlarge (lymphoblast). Each will divide rapidly forming about 400 mature plasma cells within four days. These plasma cells produce gamma globulin antibodies at a rate of 2000 molecules per second per cell. These antibodies are secreted in the lymphatic system and then enter into the bloodstream. From blood, they are distributed all over the body, seeking antigens which have invaded the body.

This processes of plasma cell activity continues for weeks until the plasma cells die. If the antigen continues to exist in the body, these dead plasma cells are replaced by new cells. Each B lymphocyte has about 100,000 antibody molecules. Each will react with only one specific type of antigen. So when an appropriate antigen attaches to the antibody on the B cell membrane, it leads to the activation process. The same thing happens in T lymphocytes. There are molecules similar to antibodies on T cells called surface receptor proteins (T cell markers). They become activated by the invasion of one specific activating antigen.

The stimulation to the immune system may be presented to the host either from outside (exogenous microorganism, pollen, etc.) or within the body (endogenous effete cells, transformed cancer cells, etc.). Hyperthermia with turbulent body fluid flows and heat makes many of the antigens and antibodies freed into blood and lymph circulation. This will result in intense stimulation of immune system. Further the mild to moderate hyperthermia simulates the production of lymphocytes which play a vital role in bodies defense against the microbes, cancers, etc.

Macrophages, the Eaters of Antigen (Fig.6)

Macrophage means big eater in Greek. There are millions of macrophages present in the lymphoid tissue. Similar cells are also found in the spleen (lining venous sinuses), liver (Kupffer cells), and skin (Langerhans cells). The macrophages in the spleen swallow fragmented old red blood cells and their hemoglobin. They digest hemoglobin thereby releasing iron to bone marrow to make more red blood cells. The protein from red blood cells is converted into bile pigments. Monocytes migrate from the blood vessels to the tissues, increasing in size (up to 80 times) to become tissue macrophages. These macrophages are part of the reticuloendothelial system (RES). They play an important role in the immune defense mechanism as the body's first line of defense.

Macrophages can swallow (phagocytosis) and destroy large quantities of bacteria, virus, dead tissue, cancer cells, and other foreign particles in the tissues. Many of the macrophages lie in opposition to lymphocytes in lymph nodes and skin. This shows that they are mutually transferring material. The processes of phagocytosis, digestion of microbes and antigens and production of interlukins is enhanced by hyperthermia. That is why I recommend mild to moderate hyperthermia to HIV infected people from the very beginning. When the invading organism or antigen reaches the lymph nodes and tissues, they are swallowed and partially digested by these macrophages and passed directly to the lymphocytes. This leads to the activation of specific clones of T and B lymphocytes. These macrophages also produce a substance called interlukin-1. It promotes the growth and reproduction of specific lymphocytes.

Broad Functions of Immune System

In summary, there are three important functions of the body's immune system:

1. Its first function is defense against the invasion of microorganisms.
2. Its second function is homeostasis, which means it preserves the uniformity of a given cell type in a multicellular organism. The immune system is charged with the function of removing damaged circulatory and non circulatory cellular elements. An aberration in homeostasis results in diseases such as auto-immune diseases.
3. The third most recently discovered function is surveillance. The immune system continually monitors the recognition of abnormal cell types (for example, red cells, white cells, cancer cells, infected cells etc.) which constantly arise within the body. These mutants may be the result of physical, chemical, viral and/or bacterial insult. The immune system is charged with recognition and disposal of newly acquired configurations. Failure of this function is thought to result in malignant diseases (cancers).

The immune system's process of cleaning the body of diseases is continual. One has to starve the disease causing cells by fasting and then enhance the body's immune system by total autoimmune urine therapy (drinking urine and hyperthermia). This will allow the immune system to removes all disease causing agents and cells. This processes is facilitated by mild to moderate hyperthermia as described in chapter 1.

Antibodies (Antitoxins)

Antibodies produced by the immune system are called immunoglobulin (Ig). They are a collection of specialized proteins which combine with a specific antigen in a lock and key fashion. These are mainly produced by plasma cells and to a lesser extent by basophils as a result of specific stimulation or an attack by an antigen (immunogen). They are released in the lymphatic system. They find their way to the bloodstream as plasma proteins and are distributed all over the body.

In humans five kinds of immunoglobulin (Ig G,D,A,M,E) are found. IgG is the most abundant. By antigenic changes many other subclasses of immunoglobulin have been added (Ig G1, 2, 3, 4). Antibodies (immune bodies) act in two different ways to protect our body against invading antigens. They first directly attack the invader. Secondly, they activate the complement systems. The production of antibodies, their circulation, and their function is enhanced by mild to moderate hyperthermia and AUT.

How Antibodies attack Antigens and Toxins

There are multiple antigen sites on invading agents. Antibodies can attack an invading agent by:

1. **Agglutination:** invading agents are bound together in clumps by antibodies.
2. **Precipitation:** soluble antigen and antibodies mix with each other and make large insoluble precipitates (like putting lemon into warm milk).
3. **Neutralization:** antibodies cover toxic sites of the antigenic agent, neutralizing their toxic effect.
4. **Lysis:** some potent antibodies directly attack the membrane of the cellular agents (bacteria, viruses cancer cells etc.), rupturing the cell membrane resulting in their death. Most of the protection by antibodies comes through the amplifying effects of the complement system described below. These activities can be enhanced by mild to moderate hyperthermia and AUT.

The Complement System

In addition to antibodies of the immune system, the human plasma (blood without cells) contains several proteins called complements. Many of the complements are enzymes. They are synthesized in the liver, in the lymphoreticular system, by the lymphocytes and monocytes. The complements are the integral part of the body immune system. They circulate in the plasma and tissue fluids in an inactive form. The complement system is responsible for enhancing and amplifying the effect of the immune defense system. Their effect is like pouring gasoline into fire.

How Does Complement System Work

When an antigen binds with a specific antibody, a portion of the antibody becomes uncovered or activated. This uncovered site will bind with a complement molecule from the plasma. This sets into motion a cascade of sequential reactions which result in formation of enzymes. These formed enzymes activate increasing amounts of proteins and enzymes resulting in a very large reaction with multiple products. These products help to prevent damage by invading organisms (antigens) and their toxins as follows:

1. Some of the products of the complement cascade activate many folds of swallowing (phagocytosis) of the antigen and antigen antibody complexes by the neutrophils and macrophages. This process results in the destruction of microbes many hundred folds.
2. The lytic (cytotoxic activity) complex of the complement cascade ruptures the cell membrane. This results in the death of viruses, bacteria, fungus, parasites, virus infested cells, cancer cells, etc.
3. Some of the complement products change the surface of the invading organism. This results in clumping of the organism (promote sticking, agglutination). This makes antigens less mobile and prevents their spread.
4. Complement enzymes and other complement products can attack the structure of some viruses making them nonvirulent (neutralization of viruses).
5. Some of the complement products cause a large number of neutrophils and macrophage to migrate (chemotaxis) into the site of insult.

Activation of Complement System

Classically the complement system can be activated by antibodies (Im, Ia), bacterial lipopolysaccharide, C reactive protein bound to pneumococci, retroviruses, heart mitochondrial membrane, polyamines, polynucleotides, urate crystals, polysaccharide (inulin), yeast cell walls, bacterial cell wall components, influenza and other viruses, fungi, certain tumor cells, cobra venom factors, nephritic factors, x-ray contrast media, and dialysis membrane in renal dialysis to name a few.

Complements and Diseases They Produce

The complement system, though tightly regulated in the body, can cause disease also. Complement activation due to recognition of autoantibodies or tissue deposits of immune complexes can result in activation of the complement. This can result in diseases such as good posture syndrome, serum sickness, hypersensitivity, pneumonitis, etc. Complement deficiencies can result in diseases such as systemic lupus erythematosus and some forms of glomerulonephritis. A complement deficiency can be congenital or acquired. Since the urate crystals and protein-polysaccharide complexes in the urine stimulate the complement system, autoimmune urine therapy can activate the complement system to combat diseases. Hyperthermia activates the complement system, its enzymes, their function.

Immune Defense Mechanisms of the Gut Wall (Fig. 5, 7)

We need to know more about the gastrointestinal (gut, intestines) tract and its role in the immune defense mechanism in order to understand autoimmune urine therapy (AUT). The small and large intestine contain hundreds of aggregations of lymphoid nodules (part of the immune system, Payers patches) embedded in the gut wall and its mesentery. They are embedded just below the absorbing surface (internal wall) of the intestinal tract in the lamina propria. This layer of intestine also contains millions of lymphocytes, plasma cells, eosinophils, and macrophages. The inner lining of the gut is thrown into finger-like projections called villi. The center of each villus in the intestine contains a lymph duct (lacteal) and blood vessels. The lacteal collects fat absorbed from the intestines and lymphocytes in a sac (cisterna chyle). This sac drains into a larger duct system called the thoracic duct. This lymph duct empties into a large vein (into the blood) on the left side of the neck. Surprisingly 95% of the lymphocytes in the lamina propria do not enter the lumen of the intestine.

Besides food, we swallow thousands of different bacteria, viruses, parasites, protozoa, fungi, spirochetes, etc. The intestines contain millions of bacteria. Some of the bacteria are helpful to the body and produce vitamins. Others can cause diseases. The large mucosal surface of the intestinal tract presents an enormous area to be protected against invasion (2,690 square feet).

The lymphoid nodules along with plasma cells, macrophage and lymphocytes (in lamina propria) form a "secretory immune system." They produce a special class of antibodies. They restrain bacterial proliferation and neutralize viruses which are entering our gut. They prevent penetration of enterotoxin through the inside wall (epithelium) of the intestine. It is estimated that the wall of the intestine contains 180,000 cells per cubic millimeter of IgA antibody producing plasma cells. In addition it contains 18,000 cells per cubic millimeter of IgG antibody producing plasma cells. There are at least 196,000 plasma cells alone per cubic millimeter in addition to other cells of the immune system. IgA antibodies are also found in the secretion of the parotid, submandibular, lacrimal, tracheobronchial, and gastrointestinal glands and in the blood serum.

When antigens pass though the intestinal wall, they are picked up by macrophages. Some of them are swallowed (phagocytosis) and destroyed by macrophages. The rest of the antigens are presented to the lymphocyte. Some of the antigens also pass the intestinal mucosal barrier and interact with cells of the lymph nodules. Some of the cells (plasma cells) come in contact with antigens and produce IgA. The other cells (lymphoblasts) of the lymph node interact with the antigens and migrate to lymph nodes in the mesentery. After further maturation, they enter the circulatory system. From the circulatory system, they return to the intestine where they are distributed in the wall of the intestine (lamina propria). Here, they differentiate into plasma cells and produce specific antibodies.

These antibodies are transposed through the intestinal lining (epithelium) and bound to the secretory component of the lining (a special glycoprotein). These specific immune glycoprotein bound complexes are released to the free surface of the intestine. They are retained on the inner surface of the gut wall (intestinal villi, glycocalyx of the epithelium). Here they react with antigens, toxins, bacteria, etc. and prevent antigen penetration of the cell lining of the intestinal epithelium. This processes is called Immune Exclusion. These lymphoid cells in the intestinal wall (lamina propria) are a barrier to the penetration of disease causing organisms and toxins from the external environment. When we drink urine, the antigens from the urine are absorbed. They are picked up by the immune defense cells in the gut wall. These cells become stimulated and start producing antibodies against the offending organism within the body. Picking of antigens and their transport to immune defense cells and production of antibodies and various lymphokines is enhanced by autoimmune urine therapy and hyperthermia.

FIGURE 5: SHOWING LYMPHATIC SYSTEM OF OUR BODY. IT PERVADE ALL CELLS AND ORGANS.
(Oval dots = lymph nodes. Thin lines = lymph channels)

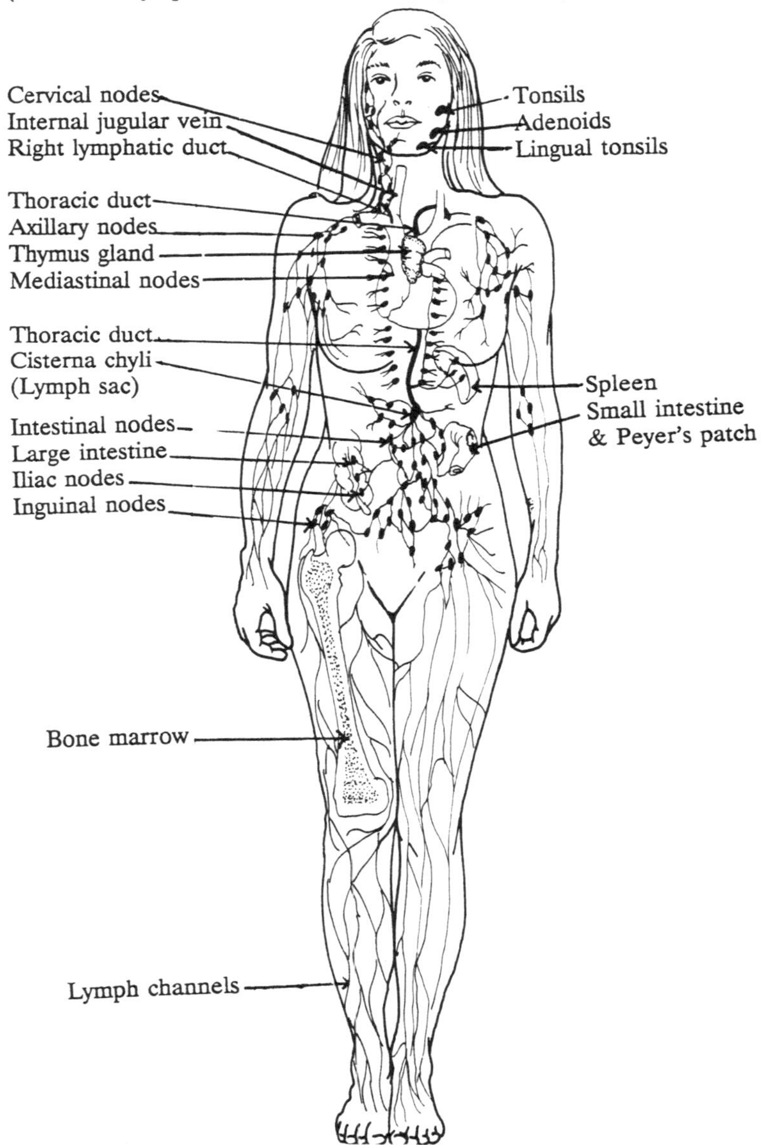

FIGURE 6: SHOWING ORIGIN OF THE WHITE BLOOD CELLS AND THEIR FUNCTION.

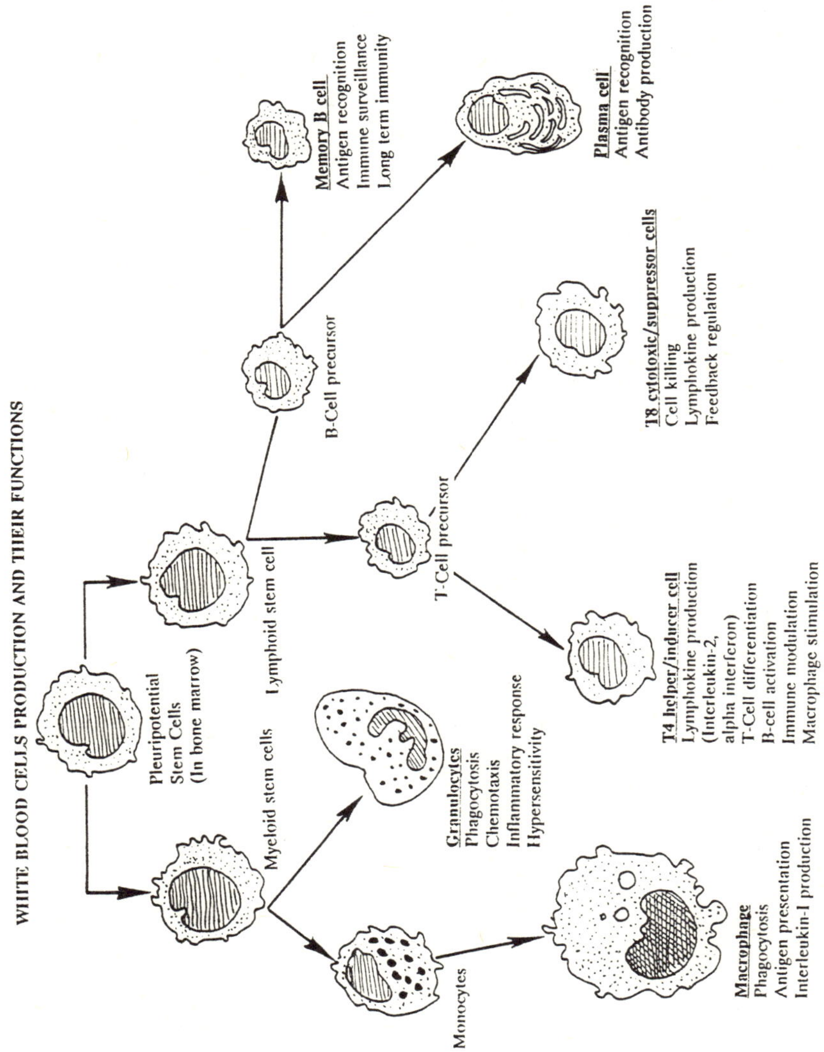

FIGURE 7: SHOWS HOW VARIOUS COMPONENTS AND ANTIGENS FROM URINE ARE ABSORBED BY THE INTESTINAL WALL, PICKED UP BY THE IMMUNE DEFENSE CELLS, DISTRIBUTED ALL OVER THE BODY.

SECTION OF A SMALL INTESTINE SHOWING THE VILLI ARRANGEMENT AND MAGNIFIED SINGLE VILLUS

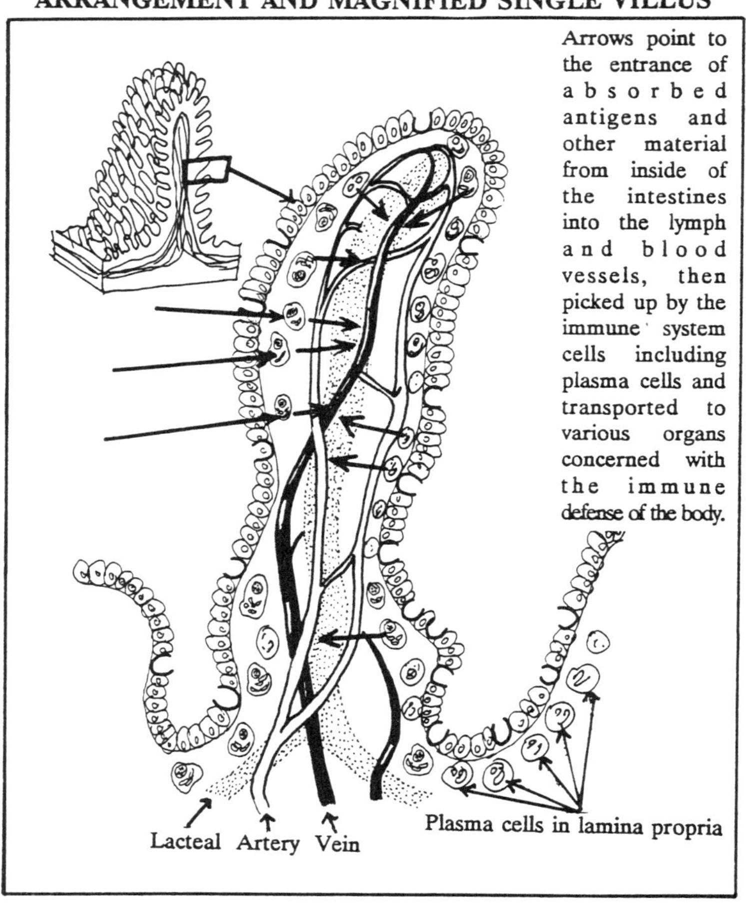

CHAPTER 9

HOW AUTOIMMUNE URINE THERAPY (AUT) AND HYPERTHERMIA CURES OR CURTAILS DISEASES

The seeds of great discoveries are constantly floating around us, but they only take root in minds well prepared to receive them.

W. B. Cannon
The Way of An Investigation

To raise new questions, new possibilities, to regard old problems from a new angle requires creative imagination and make real advances in science.

Albert Einstein

I felt sightly queasy when at lunch Francis winged into the Eagle (restaurant) to tell everyone within hearing distance that we had found the secret of life.

James D. Watson, Nobel Laureate
The Double Helix, a personal account of the discovery of the structure of DNA

To understand how urine cures diseases, we must understand how diseases are produced. There are a multitude of diseases. Their names and site of origin are irrelevant. They always arise from a foreign material such as a virus, bacteria, fungus, parasite, spirochetes, chemicals, physical forces, food, and fluid, or from substances produced within the body. These factors attack the body cells. There are an estimated 75 trillion cells in the human body. Special organs are nothing but a group of specialized cells. In a nutshell, diseases arise from an attack on the body cells by a foreign material produced within the body or by an invasion from the outside by inhalation, ingestion, contact, or injection. The only exceptions to this rule are the diseases caused by trauma, structural defects, genetic defects, and congenital anomalies.

To date, no controlled experiments have been conducted with urine in laboratory animals. Most of the literature available deals with the human experiences of conducting autoimmune urine therapy. I will explain in this chapter and other chapters why and how urine controls or cures diseases. The explanation is based on available scientific work, and my own and other people's experiences. Hyperthermia has not been tested for diseases other than cancer. Combined AUT and hyperthermia has good possibility of curing or curtailing many acute, chronic and deadly diseases.

Pasteur's Old broth: Basis for Vaccines and Immunization

Edward Jenner developed the smallpox vaccine in 1798 A.D. Almost 100 years later, in 1875, Louis Pasteur discovered a similar phenomenon while studying chicken cholera, a troublesome epidemic at that time. He isolated the organism and grew it in a broth (culture media). To maintain the active growth of bacilli, old broth was replaced with new broth at regular intervals. If the broth was not renewed, the bacilli poisoned themselves in their own waste products and died. This is similar to the way yeast cells poisons themselves from the alcohol they produce. Pasteur took a small amount of the old broth and put it in new broth to continue the growth of the bacteria. When he put a small amount of the new broth on a piece of bread and fed it to chickens, they invariably died.

During this study, by mistake, he fed the chickens with bacilli which had remained in the same broth (old broth) many days. To his surprise, these chickens did not die. Further, when these chickens were fed with active virulent bacilli from new growing broth, they still did not die. The chickens who received no pre-feeding of old broth (containing inactive bacilli) died. He postulated and proved repeatedly that the chickens coming in contact with a weakened strain of bacilli had acquired immunity. Weakened or killed strains of the bacteria did not kill the animal. Instead they produced resistance to the disease. Such an animal or subject is said to have developed immunity or is immunized or immune to the disease. He applied this principle for developing vaccines against sheep anthrax and human rabies. This opened the new era of vaccination and preventive medicine.

Typhus Vaccine Prepared from Urine

In 1942, Ludwig Fleck at a ghetto hospital in a concentration camp in Lwow utilized the urine of typhus patients as a source of specific antigenic substance in preparation of a preventive vaccine. He reported the results of his study at the staff meeting of the ghetto hospital in May 1942. Shortly after this meeting, his collaborators were exterminated by Nazis. About 500 people were vaccinated by Dr. Fleck with this urine-derived typhus antigen. Most of those vaccinated did not contract the disease. Those who contracted the typhus after vaccination recovered after a mild or abortive course of the disease. In contrast, most of those unvaccinated contracted louse born typhus, and 30% of them died of typhus. The Germans forced Dr. Fleck to produce the typhus vaccine in the camp hospitals of Lwow, Auschwitz, and Buchenwald to be used on their troops.

Tragically, Dr. Flecks family died in Auschwitz. He continued to precipitate the antigen from the urine to immunize people against typhus. His life was spared by the Nazis. He emigrated to Israel in 1957 and died in June 1961, of Hodgkin's disease (*Hospital Medical Practice*, October, 1978). This is a classic example and proves that disease causing agents such as virus bacteria, cancer cells, carcinogenic substances, and agents from many chronic diseases and their parts come out in urine. They can be used to prevent and cure diseases. AUT and Hyperthermia enhances the output of disease causing agents in the urine thus stimulates the immune system.

If these typhus patients had known of autoimmune urine therapy, they could have been healed of the typhus disease by drinking urine. The uninfected could have developed immunity by drinking the urine of patients or their own. Further, the prisoners in the concentration camps were starved. Drinking the urine would have saved them from typhus, and the ravages of starvation. Autoimmune urine therapy can be used in hunger-stricken North African countries to save millions of hungry, disease stricken children and adults. Fleck was the first to report that the white blood cells (neutrophils) become stimulated after endotoxin contact (Chemotaxis). This makes the white blood cells move faster to the site of insult, swallow bacteria (phagocytosis) quicker, and kill bacteria more rapidly.

Development of Polio Vaccine

The development of the polio vaccine is a classic example of immune therapy. The first vaccine was developed by Salk. It was composed of three antigenic variants of polio virus inactivated by formaldehyde. There were many drawbacks of this vaccine. The virus was difficult to grow, so it was difficult to provide enough antigenic mass to elicit the formation of antibodies in recipients. The degree of inactivation of the virus by formalin was difficult to control. This resulted in actual polio in early stages of this vaccination (Type III polio). To obtain the vaccination against polio, a person had to take painful shots.

Albert Sabin and his associates developed weakened strains of all three polio viruses. This vaccination is given orally on a sugar cube. These weakened viruses multiply in the gut and induce immunity. There is 1 in 2,500,000 chance of getting polio by these vaccines. A new vaccine is being developed which will not produce any polio and will be available in the USA.

Here again, AUT is not much different from the oral polio or typhus vaccine. Many types of attenuated disease-causing agents come out of urine which act the same way as the oral polio vaccine during AUT.

Types of Immunization

There are two types of immunization: active and passive. In active immunization such as in polio, smallpox, rabies, mumps, tetanus, etc., the antigen is injected or swallowed. As a result, antibodies are produced. These antibodies are constantly circulating in the body. They will attack if that particular microbe gets into the body. These antigens also stimulate clones of immune defense cells. They will multiply and produce antibodies and send an army of fighting white blood cells. This will eliminate the invading disease-causing agent and their toxic products.

In passive immunizations antitoxins are given. They work against toxins produced by the microbes. These antibodies are produced by injecting the toxins into animals. They stimulate the animals immune defense system to produce antibodies against the injected toxins. These antitoxins are extracted from the animals blood plasma. They are used in humans as a life-saving measure when a disease threatens life, such as diphtheria, tetanus, snake bites, and botulism. By injecting these antitoxin serums, the toxins inside the body are neutralized and the life is saved. Antitoxin serums, being foreign proteins from animals, can cause allergic-anaphylactic conditions. The anaphylactic reaction may result in death unless treated vigorously with epinephrine, oxygen, steroids, and antihistamines.

AUT and hyperthermia acts as both active and passive immunization. Antigens stimulates the antibody production. Antibodies, lymphokines, interferons and their broken down products act and activate similar to passive immunization. In emergency conditions, when the antivenom serum (for snake bites) and antitoxin serum (for tetanus, diphtheria, botulism, etc.) are not available, the best approach is to drink all the urine that the body produces along with plenty of water. This should be associated with fasting and can be a lifesaving measure.

Urine Effects on the Body: In Health and Diseases (Fig. 3-7)

Let us examine in detail how autoimmune urine therapy (AUT) works. I have already discussed the body's immune defense mechanism and how it defends against diseases (Chapter 7). Urine contains various parts of disease-causing agents. Parts of the various organ cells succumbing to a disease come out in the urine. The immune defense cells destroyed while fighting the disease appear in the urine. Urine also contains secretory products, the parts of the heathy body cells which are being constantly replaced by new cells, hormones, enzymes, electrolytes, and many known and unknown products (see chapter 7).

To begin autoimmune urine therapy, we start drinking all of the urine we produce, day and night, along with plenty of water. The first organ to encounter the urine is the mouth, then the back of the mouth, the gullet (esophagus), and finally the stomach. The urine dilutes the acid in the stomach. The acid in the stomach kills many living cells in the urine (viruses, bacteria, etc.). Stomach acids precipitates and denatures protein, like formalin in vaccine preparations. This acid liquid containing saliva, stomach juices, urine, and water passes rapidly to the small intestine. A small amount of urine is absorbed by the stomach. As it proceeds through the upper part of the intestine, some of the urine is absorbed along with the hormones (cholecystokinin and secretin) of the gut. These stimulate the secretions of the pancreas, bile, intestinal juices, and hormones. Urine acts as a saline cathartic (ex. Milk of Magnesia) making the pancreas and gall bladder release enzymes and bile into the intestine. Motility of the bowels is also increased. These juices are alkaline in nature and neutralize the acids and acid urine from the stomach.

Now we have the urine with all its contents, water, and all the digestive juices. These juices are absorbed back into circulation along with the urine and its contents. We know that only 40% of the urea in the urine is absorbed. The rest is passed in the stools. Thus, the gut acts like the kidneys in eliminating unwanted metabolic products. That is why there is no chance of developing toxicity by autoimmune urine therapy. Urine taken internally is expelled out of the body and is drunk repeatedly. First, it has a yellowish tinge. As the day passes, drinking urine along with fresh water and fasting results in a clearer urine output.

The urine taken orally will clean the intestines. After this, a person may have loose bowel movements. There is no cause for alarm. The loose bowel movements will stop within a couple of days. One may develop a mild, achy feeling in the head. The body will feel warmer when drinking the morning urine. Morning urine drinking should be followed with a glass of fresh water. There may be an increased heart rate due to urea content of urine. Save a portion of the urine to rub all over the body. Morning urine will be the darkest; after this, the urine will become clearer (like water) as the day passes. If the urine is darker as the day passes, it indicates that a person is not drinking enough water. If this happens, drink plenty of water(about eight glasses a day).

Antigen Distribution All over the Body (Fig.5,7)

The urine, along with disease-causing materials (antigens) and other contents, also become absorbed through the velvety wall of the intestines. The urine after hyperthermia is rich in antigens of various kinds. These antigens are denatured to varying degrees by digestive juices. Some of these antigens are already denatured by the hyperthermia treatment and become more antigenic. They are picked up by the plasma cells, macrophages, lymphocytes, and lymph nodes in the intestinal wall. These immune defense cells and lymph fluids, packed with antigenic material from the denatured disease-causing (from urine) agent, migrate to the regional lymph nodes.

The gut with its 2690 square feet of absorbing surface area, also absorbs enormous amounts of this antigenic material which enters the blood and lymph circulation through capillaries and lacteal (tiny lymph duct in the intestinal villi). From the lacteal, they enter the lymph sac (thoracic duct). They then pass on to the neck in a special lymph duct (thoracic duct) and empty into the blood circulation. From the blood circulation, they return to the intestinal wall, to all the parts of the body, to the area of disease (target organ or organs), and to all parts of the immune system. Hyperthermia facilitates this process.

Activation of Macrophages, T and B Cells (Fig.6, 7, 12)

Thus, through the blood and lymphatics, the antigens are presented to the millions of macrophages and other immune defense cells (lymph nodes, liver, spleen, bone marrow, skin, and other lymphoid tissue). These cells swallow the invading antigens, as well as micro organisms. The antigens and microbes are partially digested by macrophages. Then they are presented to the T and B lymphocytes. This results in activation of the specific clones of the B and T cells (immune defense system; see chapter 8). All these activities are enhanced by the hyperthermia treatment. That is why hyperthermia is beneficial in the treatment of chronic debilitating incurable diseases. These antigen-stimulated macrophages also secrete a substance called interlukin-I, which promotes the growth and reproduction of specific T and B lymphocytes. As long as we have disease-causing antigens coming out of the urine and we drink all of the urine produced, the immune system continues to be stimulated. The antibody production is enhanced by hyperthermia as described in chapter 1. Even mild to moderate hyperthermia also stimulates the lymphocyte production. That is why combining AUT with hyperthermia will stimulate the immune system and fight the disease. This combination could well be deadly to the AIDS, leprosy, tuberculosis, cancer, etc.

Antibody Production by B Cells (Fig.6)

Each B lymphocyte has about 100,000 types of antibodies on its surface. Each will react with only one specific type of antigen. Similarly, T cells have surface receptor proteins on the cell membrane. They are also highly specific for one specific activating antigen. There are millions of preformed clones of B and T lymphocytes. These are capable of producing specific antibodies and T cells when stimulated by a specific antigen. The B lymphocytes, with the antigen attached to the surface antibody start multiplying millions of their own clones. They start differentiating into large plasma cells and memory B cells. The plasma cells produce antibodies which attack and neutralize disease causing antigens and their toxic products. These plasma cells continue to produce antibodies in tissues all over the body for days and years until they die. Memory B cells stay in the tissue in a dormant state. They are activated to divide and produce plasma cells and more of the memory B cells as they come in contact with a specific antigen. Antibody production by plasma cells is enhanced by combining hyperthermia and AUT.

Activation of T Cells (Fig. 6, 12)

The next group of lymphocytes to be stimulated by hyperthermia and autoimmune urine therapy antigens are T lymphocytes. The antigens from autoimmune urine therapy are presented to the T lymphocytes by macrophages, blood, and lymph fluids. These antigens get attached to specific surface receptor proteins. They stimulate clones of the T cells to multiply by the millions. By antigen stimulation these T cells divide into three categories of cells (as described in the body immune defense mechanism in Chapter 7). They actively participate in cell mediated immunity. They are as follows:

1. T_4 helper inducer cells producing interlukin-II and interferon. These secretions activate the B cells and macrophages and help T cell differentiation.
2. T_8 cytotoxic cells directly attack the body cells with disease or organisms containing body cells (infected cells, cancer cells, etc.), thereby killing them. Hyperthermia activates the function of killer cells.
3. T_8 suppressor cells control the activity of T_4 and T_8 cytotoxic cells so that they will not overdo the job. The activities of all these B and T cells and macrophages have a snowball effect. Stimulation of one cell activity enhances the activity of the others.

By practicing total autoimmune urine therapy and hyperthermia, one is constantly and continuously presenting antigens to the body's immune defense system. This in turn, makes the immune system work nonstop to eradicate diseases. Constantly drinking urine is like bringing a fresh army with new equipment onto the battle field every day. Once the disease is eliminated by the heightened immune defense mechanism, the antigen output in the urine is also reduced. This results in reduced stimulation of the immune mechanism of the body. The clones of B and T cells reacting to that antigen takes rest and only become activated when the same antigen attacks the body. There are billions of plasma cells lining the wall of intestines. They come in direct contact with the antigens in urine and produce immense amounts of antibodies and related products which eradicate diseases.

Urine Therapy and Hyperthermia as Pasteur's Old Broth

Just like Louis Pasteur's discovery of the relationship between old broth and the development of immunity, fasting, hyperthermia and continuously drinking urine results in not introducing any fresh broth for the causative agent to thrive on. Reintroducing urine (along with fasting) into the body acts like an old broth inhibiting the further growth and development of the causative agents. As a matter of fact, the whole human body is nothing but a mass of culture media. Various disease-causing agents and disease-inflicted cells thrive in it.

A healthy body immune system is continuously eliminating them to maintain health. By fasting, the body becomes like old broth and the causative agents cannot thrive due to lack of new nutrients and the presence of various metabolic components, lymphokines, interferons, and antibodies. The urine contains complete living or attenuated dead causative agents or their parts, as well as the toxins and any other substances they have produced. All these components stimulate the body's immune defense mechanism the way vaccines do. Fasting with AUT and hyperthermia results in the minimal loss of antigens and antibodies from the body. They are being constantly fed back to the body. The whole immune system gets highly charged. This increases the level of circulating antibodies to the maximum, which results in the elimination of disease.

Stimulation of the Complement and Nonspecific Immune System by AUT and Hyperthermia

The urea, non protein nitrogen (NPN), urate crystals, creatinine, and hundreds of other contents in urine (see chapter 6) activate another part of the immune defense called complement system (see chapter 7). This complement system enhances the activity of the immune defense mechanisms many fold. The urea, N.P.N., creatinine and hundreds of other urinary components themselves have antiviral, antibacterial, and antitumor activity. They will act against microbes and cancer cells and end the diseases caused by them. This is proved scientifically by the injection of extracts of many bacteria (phospholipid extract of gram negative bacteria, salmonella, E. coli, cholera vibrio, BCG tuberculosis vaccine, lipopolysaccharide extract (LPS), and corynebacterium paravium) which induces resistance to numerous microbes and cancers. BCG vaccination causes regression of some of cancers (melanoma).

Autoimmune urine therapy enables the immune system to fight a specific disease. It also enhances the immune defense against other diseases because it does contain many nonspecific immune system stimulating components. Urine contains these nonspecific components in large amounts in disease states. Fasting urine and urine during and after hyperthermia contains more of these immune system stimulators than does the urine formed when a person is not fasting and heated.

Raising of the Antibody Level in the Blood

As we continue to fast and practice autoimmune urine therapy and hyperthermia, the antibody level rises higher as the days pass. There is hardly any loss of antibodies in the urine. Whatever comes out in urine is taken back into the system. The broken down antibodies which come out of urine are also absorbed from the gut. They act as the basic material to build the new antibodies. Thus, autoimmune urine therapy provides an inexhaustible supply of basic building material for antibody production. These antibodies will effectively eliminate any infecting organisms or cancers. Hyperthermia stimulates the production and release of antibodies in the body. The antibody levels in the blood will go up within 2 weeks after therapy.

Rebuilding The Body and Its Organs from Raw Material Supplied by the AUT and Hyperthermia

The human body is a collection of about 75 trillion cells. These cells are suspended in 10 gallons of body fluid. Many different organs are nothing but a collection of cells specialized to do a particular function. Every minute millions of these cells die. Death of disease afflicted cells and old cells is enhanced by hyperthermia. They are discharged through the urine, feces, and perspiration. New cells are formed to replace the dead ones. It is estimated that within two years, 90% of the cells in our body die and are replaced by new cells. Every month about 3% of our body cells are replaced by new cells. This tell us how much urine drinking can help to replenish the needed basic material derived from the dead cells and their products.

The blood, intercellular fluid, and lymph flow between the body cells, supplying the needed oxygen, enzymes, hormones, and nutrients increases especially during hyperthermia. They also remove the products of various organs and their cells and distribute them to target cells and their organs for maintaining proper functioning. Many dead cells and their metabolized parts are also moved out by these body fluids. Many cells afflicted by the disease and senile are destroyed by the hyperthermia. Thus the hyperthermia reduces the body burden of dealing with non functioning disease causing cells.

The body will have more healthy cells than unhealthy cells. It is kind of cleansing the body. Hundreds of body building materials, organic, inorganic, metabolic, non-metabolic, and complex compounds of the body secretions, come out in the urine (see chapter 7). This is specially so in the urine after hyperthermia treatment. Taking this urine back in is like replenishing the basic material for the body cells. Many of the products in urine (not needed by the body) are expelled in the stools and sweat. The remaining essential products are reabsorbed. They are used to rebuild, replace, and repair cells and maintain proper functioning.

Rebuilding and Rejuvenation of the Body

Autoimmune urine therapy at first cleanses the organs of the body. This processes is enhanced by hyperthermia due to destruction of disease afflicted cells. It relieves all obstructions in vital channels, such as blood vessels, ducts, bowels, and openings of the glands. Autoimmune urine therapy sets up a reopening process. It then starts rebuilding the organs, such as the brain, heart, lungs, liver, kidneys, endocrine glands, and immune system. This is done by reusing the wear and tear material from cells which come out in the urine. With the help of the strength given by the urine along with fasting and hyperthermia, the normal cells become very active and start using any abnormal accumulated material within their walls.

That is why I believe that the autoimmune urine therapy and hyperthermia helps in preventing further progress and reversing Alzheimer's and other chronic diseases. The cells cleanse themselves and are rejuvenated. The scavenger cells, including white blood cells, start devouring the diseased cells, and start using them for energy. This eliminates the diseased cells, non-functioning old cells, and the cells about to become cancerous. This is a kind of cannibalism at the cellular level. Hyperthermia helps to rebuild the body by removing the dead cells and their products from various parts of the body. The heat and the turbulent blood, lymph and intercellular flow created by hyperthermia helps to move these components back into circulation. Without hyperthermia, it is difficult to move and remove. Both force and heat of hyperthermia is needed to perform this function.

Hormones in the Urine

There are several hormone-producing endocrine glands in the body. They produce dozens of known and unknown hormones. Hormones put out by these glands are excreted in one form or the other in the urine. These broken down hormones are at various stages of metabolism. Traces of intact hormones are also excreted in the urine. New hormones and hormone-like substances are discovered every year from the brain and other organs. Recently researchers have discovered hormonal secretions in the heart muscle (right atrium) which are involved in heart and kidney function.

Kidneys themselves produce hormones which control our blood pressure, red blood cell production, blood thinning, and many more unknown types (see chapter 6). All these hormones are intimately involved in day to day functioning of the body. Out put of these hormones and their degradation product is enhanced by hyperthermia. These hormones and their degradation products in urine provide an unlimited quantity of basic raw material for their continued production.

Glycoproteins in the Urine

Dr. R. K. Chawla, from Emory university, reported the presence in cancer patients of a cancer-associated glycoprotein with a molecular weight of 30,000 to 60,000 daltons (JAMA, 1977, 238, p 572). It is composed of sialic acid, hexose, and hexosamine. The total amount put out in urine is 1/10,000 to 1 gram a day. This glycoprotein acts as a tool to detect cancer and its spread or remission. According to Dr. Chawla, this glycoprotein appears in urine very early. More of it is present as the cancer spreads and less of it as the cancer disappears or regresses. I believe that all cancer patients and other diseases show such glycoproteins or similar compounds in the urine.

Experiments by Dr. L. R. Stanberry and his associates have shown that the herpes simplex virus (HSV) glycoproteins have immunogenic properties. These glycoproteins can be used as immunotherapeutic agents in controlling recurrent HSV infections in humans (*J.Infect.Dis.*, 1988, 157, p.156). It is quite likely that such glycoproteins are also produced in the body and are excreted in the urine of AIDS sufferers. In the same fashion the urine of many cancer, viral, infectious, autoimmune, and other diseases contain glycoproteins which can be used to control these diseases. This is also true in HIV-infected individuals. My friends mother, an American, and her friend, suffered from herpes pain on the chest wall for many days. All the medical treatment was ineffective. This condition was promptly relieved by daily application of morning urine 3 to 4 times a day.

Hyperthermia enhances the out put of these glycoproteins. It may temporarily flare up herpes, multiple sclerosis, etc. By drinking urine every day and after hyperthermia, and applying on the external lesions, especially morning urine, one consumes these glycoproteins and microbes which are tumor and disease specific and act as antigens. Even the flare up of the diseases is short lived. They are absorbed in the bowels and picked up by the immune defense system. This results in activation of the immune system. The activated immune system will act against the cancer and eradicate it in its infancy. It is important to drink urine every day so we do not give cancer and any other diseases a chance to develop, grow, or spread.

Interferons in the Urine

Interferons (15 types of them have been identified) produced by the immune defense system, fibroblast cells and many other cells are also glycoproteins. There are three types of interferon: alpha, beta and gamma. They act by acting production of 2', 5'--oligoadenylate synthetase. This enzyme activates nucleases, and these nucleases degrade viral messanger RNA. Lack of messanger RNA results in no viral multiplication. Interferons also inhibit pathway necessary for viral multiplication such as those needed for virus adsorption, penetration, transcription, translation, assembly and release. They act on cancers such as osteogenic sarcoma, breast cancer, lymphomas, myelomas, etc. These interferons are effective in many infectious viral diseases. During AUT and hyperthermia, interferons and their degradation products which are excreted in the urine are absorbed back into the system. This boosts the body's fighting capacity against cancers, and viral and bacterial infections. Further, the broken products of these interferons act as basic building materials and help the cell to produce more interferon. Hyperthermia enhances the out put of interferons.

Free Radical Elimination by Autoimmune Urine Therapy

Autoimmune urine therapy plays an important role in mopping up all the free-floating free radicals. As discussed in the chapter on aging in the autoimmune urine therapy book (*Hyperthermia and The Water with Life*, vol. II) free radicals are produced as a byproduct of energy production in the body. Free radical output is enhanced during exercise and hyperthermia. They play an important role in the production of cancers, aging, nervous system disease, arthritis, heart and blood vessel diseases, lung disease, cataract, and many other diseases. AUT neutralizes these free radicals. The Yogis of India practice autoimmune urine therapy and live to an exceptionally old age. They do not develop any cataracts or arthritis. They have heads full of black hair, baby-like skin, and perfect mental and physical health. They can walk miles without any strain. The autoimmune urine therapy they practiced neutralizes free radicals, resulting in perfect health. Autoimmune urine therapy is the elixir of life. The explanation given as to how AUT cures AIDS (chapter 18) also applies for many other diseases.

Nature's Example: How it Handles the Discarded Material?

Let us look at what nature does with its discarded material without human intervention. For example, the luscious tropical jungles are grown on their own. How do they do it? It is simple. The dead leaves, branches, flowers, fruits, etc., of the forest and garden fall to the ground. They rot and become excellent manure. They provide all the needed nutrients to sustain plant life. This cycle repeats year after year, bringing forth abundant amounts of flowers which have the pleasing fragrances and tasty fruits.

In a similar fashion, autoimmune urine therapy makes the healthy body healthier. It restores health in a diseased body and helps us resist all infections from outside. People who practice autoimmune urine therapy are like evergreen forests enjoying a disease free status. When hyperthermia is combined, it is like combining the use of organic fertilizers with pruning a tree for healthy growth. Because the hyperthermia decreases the number of non functioning and diseased cells and disease causing antigens and microbes.

What I am trying to say here is that human beings, like all living beings, are the product of nature which surrounds us and its evolution. Why should the same principle not apply to us? Forests and gardens flourish on their own shed leaves. Urine is no different than the fallen leaves of the vegetation. Nearly ten billion cells die (0.1% of our body cells) inside our body every day. Billions of dead cells come out in the urine in one form or the other every day. The number of dead cells coming out in urine increases after hyperthermia treatment. We can flourish like beautiful evergreen forests and vegetable gardens grown naturally combining AUT and hyperthermia. The time honored concept that urine is a waste product, awful to drink, and has a bad taste should change. I cannot tell you of one scientific fact that states "this is the way urine works." There are hundreds of ways it helps the human body. It keeps the entire human body running smoothly like a well-lubricated, well-tuned engine, or like a flourishing tree in an evergreen forest.

Combining Autoimmune Urine Therapy with Hyperthermia and Chemotherapeutic Agents

I do not want to say that AUT alone will cure all the disease by itself. There is a good possibility that the autoimmune urine therapy when combined with the heating the entire body up to 38.5 to 41.8° C up to four hours and giving the drugs which are specific to a particular disease can eliminate or curtail a disease and prolong the life. The heating processes and total AUT may have to repeated many times till the disease processes is eliminated. By heating, the abnormal cells are destroyed including the causative agents. The urine produced during heating, carries with it the antigens. Feeding back such a urine will stimulate the antibody production immensely. Further, the body will get rid of all the cofactors which are responsible for stimulating the production of the disease by primary causative agents.

Heat will expose the diseased cells and the causative factors more responsive to the specific drugs. It will stimulate the immune system to attack the heat exposed causative agents and the boy cells which are affected by the disease. This method of therapy is probably more effective in diseases which do not respond well to any one method of treatment. This approach is explained in detail in Chapter 1 and 18.

Can AUT be Combined Hyperthermia and Medical Treatments?

AUT alone is effective in fighting many diseases. But it can be combined with hyperthermia, chemotherapy, radiation, antibiotics, antiviral and antifungal agents, surgery, etc. to boost the effect of AUT and increase the chances of cure. The dose of prescribed medicine need to be reduced. If a person is taking a lot of medications, a physician supervision may be needed. Because many drugs come out in the urine and drinking urine containing drugs can produce toxic reactions.

Autoimmune Urine Therapy as a Homeopathic System of Medicine

There are various systems of medicine claiming their method of treating a given disease is best. Homeopathy (G Homoios = like, similar; pathos = suffering, disease) therapy developed by Samuel Hahnemann of Germany is based on the theory that large doses of certain drugs given to a healthy person will produce certain conditions, when occurring spontaneously as a symptom of a disease. They are relieved by the same drug in small doses-- the "Law of Similia."

Homeopathy also means the prevention or treatment of a disease by a product similar to but not identical with the active causative agent (example, the Jennerian vaccine against small pox is derived from cow pox). Urine with or without hyperthermia does contain disease causing products in an altered or unaltered state. When ingested, urine acts on the disease to cure the condition as envisioned in the homeopathic principle of medicine.

AUT as Modern Medicine

Allopathy, modern medical practice, means a system of medicine in which disease is treated by producing a morbid reaction of another kind or another part. This is a method of substitution to cure the disease. Autoimmune urine therapy and hyperthermia also acts in allopathic principles. By fasting and hyperthermia, one is substituting the body's own breakdown products back into the system to heal a disease. When we use urine, we are substituting urine and its contents to heal, besides producing specific antibodies against diseases.

AUT and Other Systems of Medicine

Naturopathy and faith healing are systems of medical practice in which neither surgical or medical agents are used. Healing relies upon only non-medicinal, natural forces. Osteopathy is (osteo = bone, pathos = suffering) based on the theory that the normal human body in correct adjustment is a vital machine capable of making its own remedies against infections and other toxic conditions. AUT and hyperthermia enhances this process. The measures they use to achieve their result are natural physical, hygienic, medicinal, and surgical. A chiropractor manipulates the vertebral column to relieve pressure on nerves in the spine, so that the nerve forces can easily flow from the brain to the rest of the body. The Ayurvedic system of medicine has been practiced in India for five thousand of years. It depends mainly on herbal medicine are natural therapy to cure diseases. The modern medical system (allopathic) has many similarities to the Ayurvedic medical system. AUT embraces all these principles of medicine.

Human Body: A Pharmacological Factory (Fig. 3, 4, 7)

AUT with fasting and hyperthermia will bring back health to sick people. It is fair to say that the body is a unique pharmacological and therapeutic factory, absorbing, digesting, producing, and dispensing multitudes of biological agents such as antigens, antibodies, antisera, many hormones, hundreds of enzymes, metabolic products, glucose, protein, fats, metals, electrolytes, vitamins, blood, bone, tissue cells, organs, and many disease-causing organisms (virus, bacteria spirochetes, parasites, etc.) during diseased states. The production of above substances is enhanced by hyperthermia. These come out dissolved in the urine in liquid form. This processes is enhanced by hyperthermia. That is why it is important to combine hyperthermia with AUT. What a wonderful elixir of life, if one would only practice autoimmune urine therapy! Urine is a living water with life.

Autoimmune urine therapy encompasses homeopathic, allopathic, naturopathic, Ayurvedic, faith healing, and osteopathic systems of medicine. It is a natural product (naturopathic, Ayurvedic, and osteopathic), contains small amounts of disease-causing agents (homeopathic), other products (substitution), and other than disease-causing agents (allopathic and osteopathic).

The human body is a pharmaceutical factory producing many healing products (see Chapters 7 and 18). A person must have faith while practicing autoimmune urine therapy. There is no way any pharmaceutical company can substitute into a single product that has enormously diverse disease-healing powers that urine has. I have seen various medical disciplines claiming their system is the best in healing. Any discipline which has a good record of healing and is available to all people (rich and poor) should be used. Urine is probably the most effective, self-made, harmless, and cost-free remedy ever to emerge. It will be hard to replace this method of treatment if one would give it a chance combing with or without hyperthermia and drugs (chemotherapeutic agents).

Urine Is Truly the Water with Life and Water of Life.

CHAPTER 10

THE PRACTICE OF AUTOIMMUNE URINE THERAPY (AUT) AND HYPERTHERMIA

Guidelines

Whoever practices and teaches these commands will be called great in the Kingdom of heaven.

Matthew 5:19

Autoimmune urine therapy is discussed under two headings. The first use of autoimmune urine therapy (AUT) is to cure a disease. With this therapy one drinks all the urine with fasting and massages of urine on the skin. I call this **"Therapeutic or Total Autoimmune Urine Therapy" (TAUT)**. The next type of autoimmune urine therapy is called **"preventive or prophylactic autoimmune urine therapy (PAUT)"**. It is used to prevent the development of any disease and maintain good health. Here drink morning urine everyday and as often as one likes afterwards (at noon and evenings). Drink plenty of water and eats small amounts of food during PAUT. Combine this AUT with mild to moderate hyperthermia treatment as described in chapter 1 to cure or curtail diseases.

TAUT and PAUT

First I will discuss the process of (total) therapeutic autoimmune urine therapy (TAUT) used to cure diseases. Have determination and a will to survive and begin this therapy. Do not start AUT and give it up saying, "I can't go through with this, it does not work." Thousands of people have benefitted from AUT including myself, my family, and friends. You can do it and cure your disease. AUT is not useful for mechanical diseases like broken bones, congenital defects, and diseases.

Get a good night's rest the day before. Get up in the morning and evacuate the bowels. Brush the teeth and rinse all the toothpaste out with good clean water. Some urine enthusiasts, including myself, advise brushing the teeth and rinsing the mouth with urine. Collect all the urine in a clean glass. Drink the entire amount in one gulp without taking any breath while drinking. This method prevents aversion due to the ammoniacal smell of the urine. After drinking the entire morning urine, drink 1/2 to 1 glass of water. The morning urine has the ammoniacal smell. It has more solutes in it, tastes more bitter, and is brownish yellow to orange in color. The taste and smell of urine also depends on the type of food eaten the night before.

During total autoimmune urine therapy (TAUT), avoid food, carbonated drinks, alcohol, coffee, or fruit juices. Do not smoke or take any addictive drugs. Drink clean fresh water. As the day passes, the urine becomes more clear, has less urine smell, and becomes very easy to drink. Do not cool it, color it, or add any ingredient to change the taste. The only product that can be mixed with urine is cold fresh water and nothing else.

Continue the therapy as long as possible. There is a recorded case in J. W. Armstrong's book, in which a man practiced TAUT for 101 days, curing his blindness caused by a bee sting. He also applied the urine on his body and rubbed it on his scalp. The longer the disease (chronic diseases) exists in the body, the longer the autoimmune urine therapy has to be practiced to achieve the cure. It may take days or even months TO ACHIEVE THE CURE. Acute infectious diseases, such as pneumonia, infections, malaria, fever of unknown origin, or typhoid, etc, take less time--a few days to weeks to cure. Whereas cancers, heart and blood vessels disease, AIDS, nervous system afflictions, etc. may take 12 weeks or more of total autoimmune urine therapy combined with hyperthermia and drugs.

During PAUT, all the morning urine is ingested. During the rest of the day drink urine one or two more times. If hyperthermia is used in conjunction, all urine that comes during and after hyperthermia should be administered to enhance the immune system. Follow the guidelines as described in chapter 1. I have practiced mild hyperthermia by setting the temperature of the Jacuzzi at 105°F and staying in it without any whirlpool or water jet. The thermostat should be readjusted if the temperature in the jacuzzi has to be raised beyond 105°F.

After one week of starvation without AUT, Vitamin B group and Vitamin C deficiency may develop. After several weeks deficiency of all vitamins can develop. By drinking all the urine, hardly any vitamins or electrolytes (sodium, potassium, and chlorides) are lost. It is good to include some of these vitamins during TAUT (urine + water + no food intake). After breaking fast (one to 12 weeks of TAUT), restrict protein intake, reduce the urea output. We recommend 20-25 grams of protein a day, which is enough to maintain the body's basic needs.

Personal Experiments and Experiences

I felt a mild headache after first drinking urine, but it was gone as the day progressed. The headache may be due to excess urine output (diuresis) cause by urine drinking. After drinking urine, 40% of the urea and its related compounds are absorbed by the intestines. The urea level goes up slightly, along with creatinine and non-protein nitrogen (NPN) and electrolytes (Sodium, Potassium, Chloride, Magnesium, Calcium). All these compounds pull large amounts of water from extracellular spaces into the blood stream, causing an increase in blood volume. This increases the output of blood from the heart to all the organs including the kidneys. This increased blood flow, coupled with an increase in urea levels and electrolytes, results in more urine output (diuresis). Since water is pulled from extracellular spaces, the body cells do give up some water. This may result in reduction in the size of organs, including the brain. Because of the diuresis created by urine drinking, pressure inside the skull (cranium) also falls. This may be one of the causes for the mild headache. There may be a slight elevation of the blood pressure initially, which falls rapidly to normal or below normal.

The next effect I experienced was that my entire body felt slightly warmer, probably due to calcium and electrolyte absorption from the urine. During the first 1-5 days of UT, within 10-30 minutes after drinking urine there was a strong urge to have a bowel movement. When I went to the bathroom, I could see the old fecal material along with the urine I drank coming in a rapid surge. This kind of occurrence gradually decreased when I started drinking about a 1/2 to 1 glass of water after the urine drink. With a heavy meal the night before, this still can happen.

Within a few minutes after drinking urine, I feel and hear the churning sound in my abdomen. I can feel the rapid emptying of bile and pouring of intestinal juices. One can almost make out that mixing and churning going on inside of the gut. As noted before, only 40% of the urea is reabsorbed; the rest passes out in the feces. A good amount of Na, K, Cl, and urea is lost in the feces and sweat. Thus, there is no chance of urea accumulation in high enough quantities in the blood to cause any damage. Again, I cannot over emphasize drinking about 4-8 glasses (1200 to 3000 ml) of water a day along with all the urine. The body will not produce the needed water. If the proper amount of water is not consumed, metabolic byproducts of the cells start accumulating, resulting in toxicity to the cells and ultimately leading to death.

Fifteen cc (1/2 ounce) of water is needed to dissolve gram of solids in urine. Drink large amounts of water (4-8 glasses) to dissolve these urinary solids. When there is renal insufficiency, the functional units (nephrons, Fig. 3, 4) lose their ability to reabsorb and conserve water. Therefore, a large amount of water should be ingested to excrete the solids which come out of the kidney. During UT, morning urine is the darkest. Subsequent urine is clearer, looks almost like tap water, and is easy to drink. If urine tastes salty, reduce the salt intake and drink more water. I have observed that after entering the hot tubs and jacuzzi, and exercise, the urine is rich in antigens and tastes different. So is also the urine after hyperthermia. After mild hyperthermia in the jacuzzi, the amount of urine produced was less and was concentrated. This urine has the best therapeutic value (loaded with antigens etc.) and should never be discarded. If necessary, dilute it with water and drink it.

Drugs, Caffeinated Drinks, Hyperthermia and Autoimmune Urine Therapy

Stop taking medications during Hyperthermia and autoimmune urine therapy. If the drugs are essential, cut down their daily doses and see the effect. If there are no adverse effects, stop using the drugs. Adjusts the dose and find the dose of the drug needed. If a person is suffering from a serious illness, practice autoimmune urine therapy under the guidance of a physician. All alcoholic beverages, caffeinated and cola drinks, addictive drugs, tobacco products, betal nut and leaves, cocaine leaves, etc., are prohibited during hyperthermia and autoimmune urine therapy.

Physical and Mental Activity During Hyperthermia and Autoimmune Urine Therapy

Four to six hours of work is allowed if it does not involve strenuous physical labor. Sedentary workers can carry out their jobs without any problem. Avoid strenuous physical labor. If the person is resting at home, walking one to two miles a day is good exercise. Spend 20-30 minutes a day exercising at home. Yoga exercise are good for the body and mind. Meditation and prayers will help to soothe the mind and enhance the effect of AUT (see Chapter 20). Exercise has the same effect as mild to moderate hyperthermia. Practicing AUT, hyperthermia and exercise will have beneficial effect.

External Uses of Urine During Hyperthermia and Autoimmune Urine Therapy

Autoimmune urine therapy is incomplete without its external use. Save some of the morning urine and massage it from head to toe. It can be done one to four times a day. You need not take a bath after the external massage with urine for one to four hours. Antigens from urine are absorbed through the skin and picked up by the immune defense system cells in the skin. These cells are found all over the skin (Langerhans cells and keratinocytes) and have processes like an octopus (Fig. 10). These tentacles appear to come in contact with neighboring Langerhans cells, thus forming a continuous network in the epidermis or top layer of the skin. These cells are cousins of the macrophage. They engulf the antigen from the skin surface and present it to lymphocytes. Lymphocytes are seen surrounding them when an antigen comes in contact with these cells. These antigen loaded Langerhans cells can also move slowly to regional lymph nodes.

Thus rubbing the urine on the skin along with AUT results in stimulation of the entire body immune system. The urine and its contents act as an antiseptic, killing all the bacteria on the skin. It also opens up glandular openings on the skin, enabling the skin to breathe. It removes all the crustations. I use a soft bristle plastic brush to rub my skin and apply urine. On the beach, apply urine all over the body. It will not only prevent the bad effects of the sun, but also keeps the beach bugs away. When I first applied urine on my body, my whole skin looked like a baby's skin. Application of urine will prevent premature aging of the skin. If your are practicing AUT with hyperthermia, wait till sweating stops and then apply urine on the skin. Once the sweating stops, more urine is absorbed due to dilated blood vessels and the loosened skin layer bought on by hyperthermia.

J. W. Armstrong advocated taking seven bottles, each bottle for each day. He collected urine in each bottle each day separately. Then he began using the bottle containing seven day old urine. I do not know why seven-day-old urine is more effective for skin conditions. I have tried up to two day old urine application. Keeping urine for seven days does change the color, smell, and constituents of urine. Urine is the best skin food that exists. Apply urine on the face each morning and see the change.

Armstrong believes that autoimmune urine therapy without rubbing it externally, will result in palpitation (rapid heart beat). I see no scientific rationale for it to cause palpitations. It is caused by urea and other hormone absorption from the gut wall.

Urine Application into the Eyes, Ears, Nose, and Mouth

Besides drinking and rubbing onto the skin, the next important step is to take a dropper, fill it with morning urine, and drop it into the eyes, nose, and ears. Do not use old urine for this. Use freshly passed urine to apply to these areas. This will prevent any organism from getting into the body and enhance the local defense mechanism. Instilling the morning urine in the nose and sniffing it will prevent or reduce the incidence of colds, allergic rhinitis, hay fever, and flu. Dropping urine in the ear before swimming will end swimmer's ear infection and will clean the ears of excessive wax and infections. Urine from adults can be applied in children's ears. We practice this on our own children. If there are skin lesions, apply urine-soaked liniments. Change them every 2 to 4 hours. For mouth lesions (lips, tongue, cheek, pharynx) gargle the mouth and brush the teeth with urine as often as you can.

I have also used bottles equipped with an air pump spray to reapply urine on my body. I usually apply urine externally on my patio in warm weather and in the bathtub in winter. Heated urine packs may be applied on the mouth lesions. This regimen should be followed when a person is at home.

Can Urine Be Given Through A Vein (IV=Intravenous Route)?

Questions have been asked about giving urine through the vein directly into the blood stream, into a muscle or below the skin. Kidney failure in guinea pigs is produced by administering all the urine into the blood stream. It is useful when it is taken naturally through natural routes (oral, on skin, eyes, ears, nose). When urine is given by IV or other parenteral routes, it will not have the opportunity for its antigen to be denatured. Millions of phagocyte and lymphocytes in the gut wall lose the opportunity to pick up these antigens.

Most of the urine injected to the blood circulates back to the kidneys and is excreted as urine. Unless it is taken back repeatedly without loosing any, it looses its full effect. When given IV, the antigens are not presented to T & B lymphocytes for enhancing the immune defense mechanism. Antigen, the disease causing agent, along with toxic unwanted metabolic products are directly introduced to the blood stream. They will in turn attack the target cells in even bigger force, thus aggravating the condition. When it is given through a vein, the metabolic toxic end products which are discarded by the gut remain in the blood stream. When urine is drunk, the gut, like the kidneys, acts as the disposer of the unwanted end products of metabolism. IV use results in the toxic accumulation of these end products, thereby endangering the life.

Intravenous Administration of Urea

Urea in the body is not easily metabolized and diffuses rapidly through the kidney filter (glomeruli). Urea has been given orally or intravenously as an osmotic diuretic. Urea is given intravenously as a 10-30% solution (urevert - Travenol). IV administration causes diuresis and reduces pressure in the brain and eyes. When urea is given rapidly in the vein, it causes thrombosis, thrombophlebitis, or sloughing of the tissue due to irritation. If it is given fast (faster than 6 ml/min of 30% urea solution), it can cause nausea, vomiting, nervousness, tachycardia, and mental confusion, or raise body temperature. That is why urine should not be given through the veins, into a muscle, or below the skin. Further, it is impossible to inject the urine many times a day for many days.

Micro Allergy Clinic

William Hitts from Houston claimed that he had a legitimate doctorate degree. He opened two clinics in Houston and one clinic in Dallas Texas called Immuno Therapy and Micro Allergy clinic. He gave urine once a week for allergy and muscular dystrophy patients through the vein. The urine was centrifuged and filtered before injection and charged $80.00 /treatment. William Hitts did not have a doctorate degree and closed the clinics in accordance with the court order. Olivia Clark of Dallas testified that her son and daughter are muscular dystrophy patients received urine injections for ten weeks. They had not experienced any bouts of illness since that time (*Houston Chronicle*, 1987).

There is no way to remove all the so-called impurities from urine. During filtering, urine loses much of its healing power. If all the urine is given through IV, it will cause irritation of the vein through which it is given. It will go back to the kidneys and excrete. This can also lead to inflammation (phlebitis), thrombosis, emboli (traveling clot) formation, and toxic product accumulation, and is a threat to life. Why pay money some body when you can get better results by drinking.

How to Practice Autoimmune Urine Therapy When There Is a Mental Aversion to Drinking Urine (Fig. 8)

There are people, due to psychological or other reasons, who cannot drink urine. They have a mental block and/or are suffering from incurable or chronic diseases. For such people, urine can be administered through a nasogastric, gastrotomy, or jejunostomy feeding tubes. One can practice passing the tube through the nose or mouth. After gagging a few times, passing the tube becomes a habit and can be accomplished easily. This tube is passed into the upper part of the food pipe (esophagus). Feed the urine with the help of a syringe, funnel, medical pump which pump fluids, or through an intravenous drip bottle attached to the nasogastric and other feeding tubes. Follow it with water feeding through the same tube or drinking. Remove the nasogastric tube before going to bed and reinsert it in the morning. The following diagrams show various tubes that can be used to feed the urine.

AUT for Those Who Cannot Drink or Eat Due to Diseases (Fig. 8)

For those who cannot eat or drink at all due to diseases of the nervous system, mouth, larynx (wind pipe), esophagus (food pipe, gullet), inside the chest, heart and its blood vessels, lungs, stomach, liver, etc., there is a way of administering urine and water. These extremely ill people can have gastrostomy or jejunostomy tubes inserted through the wall of the upper abdomen and into the stomach or small intestine (jejunum) by a surgeon. These tubes can be left for long periods of time without causing any ill effect. The urine, nutrients, and any additional medications are fed through these tubes. Many of these sick and debilitated patients have catheters inserted into the bladder (Foley's catheter) and urine is collected into a bag. In such cases, when 8 ounces of urine (one glass) collects in the bag, recycle it back through the above described tubes or give it to drink. There are small medical pumps which can also be used to feed the urine from the urine collecting bag into a feeding tube every 4 to 8 hours. If a person is undergoing surgery, feed all urine produced under anesthesia and during surgery. See the given diagram in this chapter.

Methods Used to Collect Urine during Monthly Periods in Women

During the monthly periods, urine is sometimes mixed with menstrual blood. To collect urine during monthly periods, clean the genital outlet with a clean wet towel or with clean warm water. Separate the two labia with the fingers, then passes the urine directly into a glass.

Outlines of Instructions to Follow for Therapeutic (Total) Autoimmune Urine Therapy (TAUT)

1. Rest completely.
2. Wash your face and brush your teeth with urine.
3. Collect all urine in a clean glass; save enough to be used externally, and drink the rest completely. If patient is unconscious or under sedation during hyperthermia, administer all the urine back through a feeding tube.
4. After drinking urine, drink water.
5. Use the remaining urine to apply to the nose, ears, and eyes. Gargle the mouth with leftover urine, and brush the teeth with urine.
6. Collect some urine in a bowl and apply it on your body (head to toe). Rub it all over your body thoroughly up to an hour at a time 3 to 4 times a day.
7. Do not smoke or drink any acholic or nonalcoholic beverages or take any additive drugs. Do not eat any food.
8. Continue this therapy till the disease is cured or curtailed. If you can tolerate this therapy, practice it for one to three months.
9. If there are lesions on the skin or month, apply urine soaked liniments. Keep applying it till the condition is healed.

10. After total autoimmune urine therapy, start eating mild, nutritious food. Do not over-indulge. Breakfast with fruit juice. Follow total autoimmune urine therapy with prophylactic autoimmune urine therapy.
11. Drink all the urine during and after mild, moderate or severe hyperthermia to enhance the effectiveness of TAUT.
12. Repeat TAUT after PAUT if the disease condition is not eradicated or brought under control. Combine the AUT with hyperthermia as described in chapter 1.

Instructions to Follow for Prophylactic Autoimmune Urine Therapy (PAUT)

1. Requires physical and mental rest with 30-60 minutes exercise of your choice (walking, cycling, jogging, tennis, swimming, jazzercise, etc.). Follow the exercise regimen during PAUT also.
2. Maintain proper bowel movements and urine output by eating mostly vegetables diet and drinking plenty of water.
3. Take mild baths.
4. Do not eat bulky meals. Avoid spicy, salty, fatty, oily, and fried foods.
5. Do not eat until you are hungry.
6. In early stages of the disease, undergo mild to moderate form hyperthermia followed by urine therapy during and following hyperthermia.
7. Expose the body to proper sunlight.
8. Practice total autoimmune urine therapy once a week.
9. Drink morning urine along with a glass of water. Drink some more urine at noon and at evening time.
10. Do not stay awake all night or spend time on unnecessary activities.
11. Drink all the urine during and after going through the hot sauna, hot tub, jacuzzi and exercise. It ia an excellent source of antigens.

FIGURE 8: DEPICTIS VARIOUS METHODS OF URINE FEEDING IF A PERSON CANNOT DRINK.

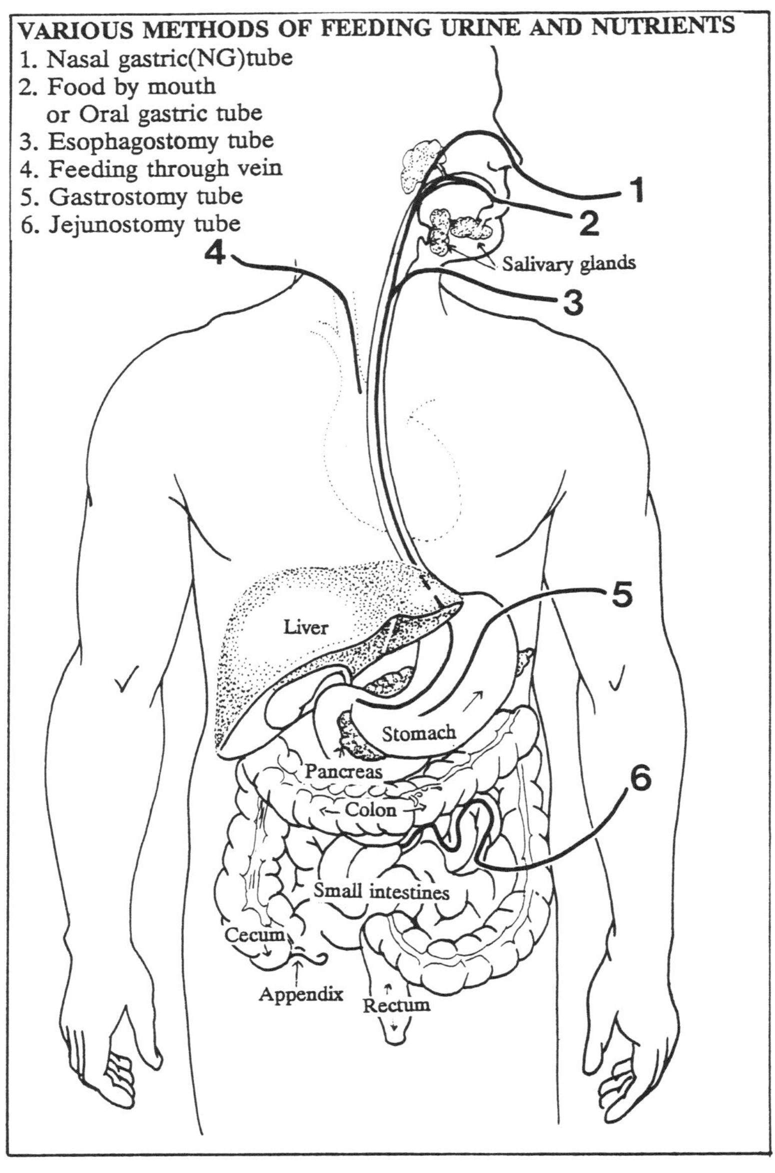

CHAPTER 11

FASTING DURING AUTOIMMUNE URINE THERAPY AND HYPERTHERMIA

Blessed are those who hunger and thirst for righteousness, for they shall be satisfied.

Matthew 5:6

Reasons for Fasting during Autoimmune Urine Therapy and Hyperthermia

Fasting along with autoimmune urine therapy (AUT) and mild to moderate hyperthermia is very important. According to the Bible, "Whenever you fast, do not put a gloomy face as hypocrites do, . . . Truly I say to you they have their reward." (Matthew 6:16). Practice fasting with autoimmune urine therapy with a good feeling and cheerfulness. This will add psychological benefits to the healing process (see Chapter 20). Do not practice AUT with disgust, out of compulsion, and/or while expressing distress. Such a mental attitude will reduce the befits of AUT.

The reasons for fasting are many. Almost every physician recommends body rest during and after illness. As in physical rest, organs such as the intestines, kidney, liver, endocrine glands, brain, skin, and all other organs in the body need what I call "chemical rest." During fasting all these organs do not stop working completely. Fasting will reduce their activity. This gives time to rebuild, repair, and rejuvenate worn out parts. Urine acts as a natural hunger suppressor. It acts by increasing the cholecystokinin and secretin production and absorption. These hormones stimulate the secretion of digestive enzymes. In addition, cholecystokinin inhibits stomach motility, thereby inhibiting hunger pains. One does not feel the craving for food which is very common in fasting without AUT. This is one of the reason why AUT is excellent for reducing weight. The normal human body produces 1200 ml of saliva, 2000 ml of stomach juices, 1200 ml of pancreatic enzymes, 700 cc of bile, and 2100 ml of intestinal secretion. With fasting, the production of these digestive enzymes is reduced. This will give rest to the organs which produce digestive enzymes and hormones, thus allowing time to repair wear and tear.

Fasting and Its Effect on Fecal Matter

The feces normally contains 75% water and 25% solid material. The solids are composed of 30% dead bacteria, up to 20% fat, up to 20% inorganic matter, 3% protein, and 27 to 30% undigested roughage. The brown color of the feces is due to bilirubin from the liver (stercobilin and urobilin). The odor of feces comes from bacterial activity in the colon and from the food we ate (indole, skatol, mercaptan, hydrogen sulfide).

AUT with fasting completely cleans the gut wall. It removes all the old decal matter sticking to the wall within 3-5 days. Fasting results in minimum feces production. The urine and its contents are absorbed completely (Fig.7). Urine will not be diluted by existing fecal matter and food material we would have eaten. Thus by fasting, we obtain maximum beneficial effects of autoimmune urine therapy and hyperthermia.

Complete Cleaning of the Entire Gut (Intestines)

Urine cleans all the fecal remnants in the gut. The cells lining the wall of the gut are shed off every three to six days, and the entire intestinal lining is replaced within one week. All the intestinal lining is not shed off in one mass at one time like a snake's skin. Every hour, thousands of cells are shed at different sites and replaced by new cells. In one week of autoimmune urine therapy, the urine and its content come in direct contact with a new cell lining of the 2690 squire feet of absorbing gut wall. There is mo more food coated intestinal lining left. Because of fasting, many of these shed cells are digested by the gut's digestive juices and used as nutritive material. This is like the leaves which fall under the tree, rot, and provide nutrients for the tree. The same cycle repeats here. With fasting and using AUT, the turnover of these cells is slowed down. It takes a long time to renew them, thus reducing the number of multiplication of the lining cells of the gut. The reduction in the rate of cell division results in a lower chance of it becoming cancerous. Thus autoimmune urine therapy reduces the chances of gut cancer.

Unless the bowels are properly scoured, the lining of the intestine (villi) is coated with old fecal matter. It gets absorbed into the blood and lymphatic systems, causing toxic effects. I have seen hundreds of surgical procedures with gut irrigation. No matter how well it is cleaned with water, it still has a coating of fecal matter. Meat, white bread, sweet danish, donuts, and well boiled processed vegetables are examples of food that cling to the bowels. Whole meal bread, bran, grapes, raisins, figs, and vegetables (celery, carrot, steamed beans, etc.) have cellulose or roughage which increases the bulk inside the gut and removes the old fecal matter coating the lining of the intestines naturally. Offensive stools and flatus are signs of old stool coating the bowels. Repeated cleansing with high enemas will not clean the 2690 square feet of absorbing gut wall completely either. Total autoimmune urine therapy with fasting serves the purpose of cleaning the bowels completely in less than a week.

Reduction of Urea Production and Giving Rest to the Kidneys

Four grams of protein produce one gram of urea. Fasting reduces the amount of urea produced and excreted in the urine. This gives rest to the kidneys. Fasting urine has less urea, and less urea is absorbed when such urine is drank. After a heavy night meal, the urine passed the next morning is rich in urea content. It is deep yellow in color, has an ammoniacal odor, and is somewhat bitter to taste. During mild to moderate hyperthermia the urea content of the urine is high. On the other hand, with severe hyperthermia with proper fluid balance, the urea content of the urine is reduced.

Effect on the Intestinal Bacterial Content

Laboratory experiments show that protein starved animals exhibited lower incidence of bacterial spread systemically from the gut to other organs compared with other animals. Starvation or protein malnutrition increased levels of gram negative enteric bacilli in the caecum (beginning of the large intestines, Fig. 8). It decreases the levels of lactobacillus and strict anaerobes (*Arch Surg*, Vol 22, Sept., 1987). Combining the autoimmune urine therapy along with fasting will reduce the entire flora of disease-causing (pathogenic) bacteria in the gut wall. It cleans all the fecal residue attached to the walls of the gut and brings back the harmony. Hyperthermia also reduces the disease causing bacterial content of the gut.

There are many bacteria present in the absorbing proximal part of the colon. They produce Vitamin K, B12, thiamine, riboflavin, etc., and gas (flatus) in the colon. The distal colon functions as a storage for feces and a residence for millions of bacteria. The absorbing proximal colon also secretes bicarbonate ions which help to neutralize the acidic end products of the bacterial action in the colon. By fasting with autoimmune urine therapy, the colon allows all these bacteria to function properly and their end products, vitamins, to be absorbed efficiently.

Energy Production in the Body

Fats, glucose, and protein are broken down in the gut and enter the cells as fatty acids, glucose, and amino-acids. They are used in the cell's powerhouse, the mitochondria, by a series of enzyme activities that produce adenosine triphosphate (ATP). ATP is a protein containing adenine, ribose sugar, and a phosphate radicle. The ATP, like gasoline for an engine, is the intracellular storehouse of energy and is used for: (a) the membrane transport of Potassium, Calcium, Sodium, Chloride, Hydrogen, phosphate, urate, ions, and many other special substances; (b) synthesis of chemical compounds, protein, phospholipid, cholesterol, purines, pyrimidines, and a host of other substances including secretions of glands; (c) mechanical work - body movements, muscle contraction, heart pumping, biliary motion, phagocytosis, ameboid movement, etc.; and (d) absorption of food from the gut. Many hormones such as insulin, steroids, epinephrine, and growth hormone play a major role in the metabolism of fats, glucose, and proteins and production of energy, ATP.

Effects of Fasting on Glucose, Fats, and Proteins

The human body is made up of 20% fat and 20% proteins. These reservoirs can provide two to three months' supply of energy during fasting. Carbohydrates are stored as glycogen in the liver (70 grams) and in muscle (200-400 grams) and body fluids (20 grams). The body has a one day supply of glucose. There are fat depots but no protein depots. Most of the protein is in the muscles and the organs (gut, brain, kidney, liver, plasma, white blood cells etc.). During fasting, all glucose stores are used in one day. The major effect of fasting after one day is depletion of fat and protein. Fat and proteins are the source of energy. Their use and depletion continues unabated. By the sixth week of fasting, most of the body fat reservoirs are used up. First there is rapid depletion of proteins during the first two weeks of fasting. Then depletion is slowed down till sixth week. At this time rapid loss of proteins starts again.

There are reports of fasting with autoimmune urine therapy for up to 101 days without any ill effects. Death results when 50% of the body proteins are used up. Hyperthermia does creates a kind of heightened fasting effect due increased metabolism. But drinking urine will spare the proteins and the body fats are used for energy. That is why AUT with or without hyperthermia is one of the best way to reduce wight without upsetting any body function (physiologically).

During fasting, glucose is formed by converting protein in the liver (gluconeogenesis). It is used mainly by the brain. As the readily available proteins are used up, the remaining proteins are hard to remove. Thus the conversion of proteins into glucose drops by almost 80%. The decreased availability of glucose through protein conversion results in rapid fat mobilization from fat stores leading to ketosis (acetone, acetoacetic acid, beta hydroxy butyric acid). These ketone bodies derived from fat and proteins enter the brain and are used as energy instead of glucose. Many of the ketone bodies also come out in the urine. During hyperthermia, the production of ketone bodies is lower than expected because, the cell burn the ketone bodies and product of fat breakdown efficiently due to increased enzyme activity in the cells due to heat.

Any excess fat is stored in fat depots. Excess glucose is converted into fat and stored. During severe hyperthermia, due to intense cell activity and increased metabolism, most of the sugar in the cells gets used very fast. That is why we gave glucose intravenously to maintain proper tissue energy needs to our cancer patients. When the tissues fill their quota of protein, the excess protein is converted into fat and stored. Proteins can be broken down and converted into glucose or fat. Glucose can be converted into fat and not protein. Those who indulge in excessive amounts of protein or carbohydrates become obese due to their conversion into fat.

Urine as Nutrient and Protein Saver during Fasting

Look at the list of nutrients, urine contains amino acids, fats, carbohydrates, electrolytes, hormones, metals, enzymes, etc. (see Chapter 7). During hyperthermia the urine contains more of these substances. When fasting with AUT and hyperthermia, the depletion of protein is reduced. The urine contains many nutrients, including ketone bodies. They are absorbed from the digestive tract and used for energy needs. AUT, like carbohydrates and fats, spares the breakdown of protein for energy. Along with fats and carbohydrates, the urine can be called a "protein sparer." Fats are used for energy. This reduces the fat deposits, resulting in loss of body weight. That is why total autoimmune urine therapy along with mild to moderate hyperthermia is the best and harmless method of reducing excess body weight (obesity). AUT acts by reducing fat stores and sparing proteins.

Fasting During Hyperthermia

Feeding back urine during hyperthermia helps to prevent breakdown of protein stores. Many heat denatured proteins derived from cancer cells and disease causing agents are fed back. These proteins act as excellent protein spares, and antigen stimulating the immune system. Practice total urine therapy with fasting for 2-3 days before hyperthermia. This will clean the entire intestinal track. It will allow the intestines to absorb all the antigenic material produced during hyperthermia without getting mixed up with old fecal matter.

Precautions to Take after Breaking the Fast

After breaking the fasting with autoimmune urine therapy, go easy on foods. Do not get into the habit of eating sugars, coffee, tobacco, carbonated drinks, etc. Eat small balanced meals containing proteins, carbohydrates, vitamins, minerals, and fiber. Avoid animal fat. Use fresh vegetables, unsalted nuts, skimmed milk, and steamed vegetables. Avoid using salted, canned, preserved, and frozen foods. Use fish for protein. My second choice is chicken or turkey. Avoid red meat or use lean cuts. Avoid hamburger meat (high in animal fats). Essential proteins needs can be obtained from a soy bean product called tofu and lentils. Buttermilk and yogurt (curds) prepared at home are also an excellent source of proteins.

After breaking the fast, continue to drink morning urine along with water all your life. This will act as prophylactic therapy against any future diseases. J. W. Armstrong drank all the urine he passed for nearly 27 years without any ill effects. Urine is not your enemy. "It is a water of life and water with life." Supplement the drinking of morning urine with one to three times additional urine drinking during the rest of the day. Whenever possible, practice total autoimmune urine therapy along with rubbing urine all over the body. This will keep your body young, disease free, and mentally fit.

During prophylactic AUT do not eat heavy, rich, bulky meals. Your diet should contain rice, potato, fruits, vegetables, legumes, brans, and yogurt in proper proportion. When the kidneys are functioning normally, it takes about 800 cc of urine to dilute and excrete 50 grams of solutes. In diseased states, it requires 3000 cc of urine to excrete 50 grams of solutes. With the usual diet, urine contains 50 grams of solutes. While fasting, this output is reduced to 40 grams or less. With a 100 gram carbohydrate diet, only 20 grams of solutes are put out by the kidneys. Carbohydrates are an efficient fuel and are burned well, with the least amount of metabolic products in the urine.

Very Sick People and Fasting

For those who are very sick and debilitated, total fasting should be avoided. Eat small amounts of nutritive meals along with plenty of fruits, vegetables, and vitamins. The very sick should be started on prophylactic autoimmune urine therapy (PAUT) combined with total urine therapy as described before. Practice autoimmune urine therapy and hyperthermia under the guidance of a physician if a person is very sick and debilitated. If hyperthermia is needed, they may not tolerate 2-3 hours of severe hyperthermia therapy. Depending on the condition of the patient mild to moderate hyperthermia may have to be practiced. Once TAUT is completed, combine PAUT, and along with TAUT, for a week or two along with mild to moderate hyperthermia. Continue this practice all through life. This will maintain a **disease-free, doctor-free drug free, debt free, worry free body and mind.**

CHAPTER 12

HOW LONG IT TAKES FOR AUTOIMMUNE URINE THERAPY (AUT) AND HYPERTHERMIA TO CURE OR CURTAIL DISEASES

A time to kill and a time to heal,
A time to tear down and a time to build,
A time to tear and a time to mend,

Ecclesiastes 3:3,7

When glandular cells (salivary gland, tear glands, pancreas, stomach, intestines, endocrine glands, etc.) are stimulated to produce proteins, newly-formed protein molecules can be detected at the maturation site of cells (the Golgi apparatus) within 20 minutes. They are secreted from the surfaces of the cells within one hour. This shows how fast the activity in a cell can be initiated. Such an activity is seen in the glandular cells, which produce various enzymes and hormones in the body (exocrine and endocrine glands). Most of these glands have pre-formed secretory material inside their cells. They can release these secretory materials on demand and instantaneously. Hyperthermia enhances the formation of secretions, antibodies and lymphokine production instantaneously. That is why combining hyperthermia with AUT results in attacking the disease immediately.

Similarly, the body's defense mechanism starts attacking the foreign material (bacteria, virus, or any antigen) within minutes of its contact. It may take two to four days to secure all its forces to come to the rescue and fight. It may take days to overcome the invader. Hyperthermia increases the circulation of all the body fluids. The movement of substances in and out of the cells and tissues is also enhanced. This results in moving the immune defense forces close to the site of insult. This is one of the important benefits of hyperthermia besides other discussed benefits in chapter 1. If the immune defense system fails to overcome the invader, the body finally succumbs.

Division of T and B Cells by Antigen Stimulation

Each B lymphocyte (white blood cells) has bout 100,000 antibody molecules on its outer wall. It will react specifically with one specific antigen. When the proper antigen comes along, it attaches to the cell membrane immune defense cells. These cells differentiate rapidly into plasmablasts and lymphoblasts which mature into antibody producing plasma cells and cell-attacking lymphocytes. **Within four days, 400 to 500 antibody producing plasma cells are produced from one single plasmablast.** The mature plasma cell produces the gamma globulin antibodies at an extremely rapid rate of about 2,000 molecules per second per cell. These antibodies enter the blood, and lymphatic fluids and are distributed throughout the body. This process continues for several days to weeks until the death of the plasma cell. T lymphocytes also divide, producing millions of clones of T cells in response to the antigen. They in turn attack the disease causing agents (antigens) and disease infected cells. Hyperthermia enhances the production and activity of T & B cells. After hyperthermia, the number of healthy young T cells increases. So AUT is very beneficial when combined with hyperthermia. It acts as a natural stimulator of immune defence cells.

Antibody Production

Gamma globulins, called immunoglobulin, are the antibodies. They have 150,000 to 900,000 molecular weight. They make up about 20% of the plasma proteins. There are millions of such clones of plasma cells produced, which put out huge amounts of antibodies to fight the disease. A single plasma cell can produce its weight in antibodies within a few days. A phagocyte (macrophage) can swallow a single bacteria or antigen in less than 1/100th of a second. This activity is enhanced many folds by hyperthermia. Then the white blood dells are actively gobbling and digesting organisms and disease infected cells.

Autoimmune urine therapy has its effects on the secretory glands of the body as soon as it is ingested. Then it starts acting on the other systems. Within one week, the immune system is at its maximum activity and the antibody production reaches its peak by the middle of the second week (11th day). The local effect on the entering organism is almost immediate (local reaction of inflammation--redness, pain, swelling, hot to touch). This is caused by white blood cells trying to localize and eliminate the offending agents. This will prevent the spread of the organism to the other parts of the body. Controlling and localizing an infection at the site of entry is an important immune defense mechanism. As millions of new plasma cells are produced due to hyperthermia, they putout large amounts of antigens. Feeding large amount of antigens produced during hyperthermia also enhance the production of disease fighting antibodies.

Besides special clones of B and T lymphocytes, other types of white blood cells are produced in response to antigens introduced by autoimmune urine therapy and hyperthermia. The longer the body had the disease, longer the autoimmune urine therapy and hyperthermia take to get rid of it. Infectious diseases are cured with short periods of autoimmune urine therapy and hyperthermia. Chronic illnesses, especially cancers, arteriosclerotic diseases, adult diabetes, AIDS, lupus erythematosus, leukemia, multiple sclerosis, leprosy, etc., may take months of total autoimmune urine therapy and hyperthermia before they are cured. I do believe that the repeated hyperthermia along with AUT with or without anti leprosy drugs may cure the disease much faster with least neurological and physical defects. If a skin lesion is present for some time, it may take days or weeks of urine application to achieve the cure. For example, superficial burns and poison ivy will take a week to heal. Itching stops within minutes and blister formation in hours. Whereas, eczema, lupus, psoriasis, Kaposi's sarcoma, leprosy, etc., take a long time to achieve a cure. The persistent practice of AUT will prevent and cure a disease in its own time.

CHAPTER 13

WHY DRINK YOUR OWN URINE?

Auto or Self Autoimmune Urine Therapy

Animals are equal, but some animals are more equal than others.
George Orwell

46 Chromosomes and 46 Million Genes in each Cell in our Body

There are 75 trillion cells in the human body. Every cell in the human body holds an intricate chemical blueprint called a gene (life molds) which guide all growth and development. These chemical blueprints are housed inside the cell's nucleus. They are made up of 46 chromosomes. Each chromosome holds at least one million genes. These genes are made up of more than three billion chemical base pairs, which are the code of life. So far, scientists have located 1,500 human genes and mapped the chemical sequence in some of these genes. It would take a 3 billion dollar program to decipher the entire human genetic code. Such a project could explain how human beings develop from a single cell. It could prepare the way for the treatment or cure of more than 3,000 inherited diseases such as Huntington's disease, cystic fibrosis, polycystic kidney, muscular dystrophy, sickle cell anemia, manic depression, etc.

Uniqueness of Each Individual

Peter Medawar, a Nobel Prize winner in medicine, pointed out in his book, *The Uniqueness of Individual* (London, Methuen &

Co., Ltd, 1957), that "the difference between individual combinations or as mathematicians say, combinational differences; one individual from all others, not because he has unique endowments, but because he has a unique combination of endowments." The endowments he refers to are genes.

J. D. Ebert in his article in the book, *The Cell* (Academic Press, N.Y., 1959, vol. 1), on the acquisition of biological specificity noted, "The difference between two individuals . . . of specific molecule not restricted to certain tissues but common to all or most all of the parts." Except for identical genotypes (identical twins), each individual is different from all other individuals and from all other organisms. So is also the urine we produce. These differences are due to the genes in our cells. With the help of our genes, the cells in our body synthesize and reproduce cells of their own type, respond to internal or external stimuli, repair damage, and defend and protect against attack. Genes are the key to the cell's function and in turn the human body.

So the organisms of different species and various individuals belonging to the same species possess a unique chemical, biochemical and biological identity (except the genetically identical twins). Macromolecular constituents of their cells, body fluids, and the protein complexes body cells produce, as well as the urine have different biochemical compositions. The immune system protects the individual from exogenous macromolecules such as viruses, microorganisms, cells, or any macromolecule which does not agree with the body. It also acts as a security gatekeeper (surveillance) whereby no foreign material is introduced by endogenous organs. Hyperthermia with AUT actually eliminates any foreign material introduced from within or from outside.

Immune System and Foreign Configurations

Lymphocytes have the ability to recognize macromolecules (antigens) and various micro organisms, as well as cells which have a chemical pattern different from the normal constituents of the individual they inhabit. They can set a specific defensive reaction to eliminate such invaders. This is called the primary immune response. During their life span lymphocytes arise continuously, each genetically programmed to respond to a single antigen. When that antigen comes in contact with such a cell, that particular lymphocyte divides (clones) and proliferates. This results in an increased population of effector cells, lymphocytes, and plasma cells, which dispose of foreign configurations. Then some memory cells revert to an inactive state, and have the capability of setting an immune response with greater efficiency when they encounter that specific antigen again (secondary immune response). This is the basis for vaccines such as tetanus, diphtheria, polio, measles,etc.

It is important to note that the introduction of bacteria, viruses, or any other foreign proteins (nonidentical) from another person into the body leads to the alteration of synthesis of some protein of the host (recipient) by lymphocytes.

Body cells and their defense system are set to their own way of reacting and relating to each other. By drinking our own urine, we are not introducing a new challenge to the already diseased body. The urine of another person may not contain the broken down or intact macromolecule (antigens) which are causing the disease in the person who is drinking the urine. The immune defense systems will have to spend their energy to fight the new macromolecule (antigens) introduced from someone else's body. Due to the lack of these disease-causing antigens in the urine from another person, their urine will not cure the disease in another person. As the saying goes, "diamonds cut diamonds"; so also is your own urine for your own diseases.

Fasting and hyperthermia will also prevent the strain bought on by foreign configurations. Hyperthermia will enhance the destruction of old and disease affected cells in short time better than most processes we know. Hyperthermia and AUT cleans the entire body of any foreign configurations, and let the immune system recuperate, rejuvenate, and function to the fullest capacity.

Urine of Other People, Identical Twins, and Animals

To cure a disease, one has to drink his/her own urine which contains many or all of the components of the disease-causing macromolecule (antigens). The urine of another person can be drunk only in (homozygous) identical twins suffering from the same disease. Urine of another person can be used locally in adults and children. Drinking cow's urine, as indicated by J. W. Armstrong, is even of lesser value. It may have prophylactic effects by its own right (orally taken or externally applied) but is of less effective when used to cure a specific disease.

The only situation where someone else's urine can be used temporarily is when there is no urine output at all from the kidneys. Until urine flow is established one can drink another person's urine. Once the urine flow begins, practice auto (self) autoimmune urine therapy. Also, someone else's urine can be used externally temporarily.

Organ Transplants and the Immune System

Use of our own urine is well exemplified by the heart, lung, liver, kidney, pancreas, and other organ transplants. If the body tolerated these and other organs from any or everybody, we would be removing the healthy organs from the dying and implanting them to replace diseased organs. This could save thousands of lives. Even now, with all our advances, we can name the organs which can be successfully transplanted from another person. Those who have undergone an organ transplant take medications to suppress the immune system; otherwise, the new organs will be rejected. Even with immune suppression, many of the transplanted organs in the host are rejected with the passage of time. Persons who can donate an organ without the fear of rejection are identical (homozygous) twins.

Urine as an Organ

In the above fashion, the urine is almost like an organ. One has to drink one's own urine to get the benefits. Drinking someone else's urine will only create hostility in the body without any benefits, such as organ rejection. Auto (self) autoimmune urine therapy is biologically, physiologically and disease specific. Because each individual has a unique combination of endowments and its associated diseases. Do not contaminate these endowments and diseases with someone else's urine.

Effect of Hyperthermia on Foreign Configurations

With AUT has a way of cleaning the entire body. Hyperthermia denatures many foreign configurations and excreted through kidney. When they are fed back, they can act as antigens producing antibodies which act against the foreign configurations. Thus hyperthermia combined with urine therapy eliminates all most all the proteins with the foreign configurations within the body which cause cancers, infectious diseases, autoimmune disease and other diseases. By eliminating most of the foreign configurations, the immune system is free to deal with the body defense effectively. This is another method how hyperthermia acts synergistically and helps to eliminate diseases and keep us healthy.

CHAPTER 14

EXTERNAL USE OF URINE AND SKIN HYPERTHERMIA

On Skin and Mucous Membranes

But when you fast, anoint your head and wash your face.
Matthew 6:17

Wash yourselves and make your self clean.
Isaiah 1:16

Structure of the Skin

Knowledge of the structure and function of the skin is needed to understand how it works in health and disease. The human body is covered by uninterrupted layers of cells called skin. The skin measures about 1.8 square meters (21 square feet compared 2690 square feet of absorbing gut wall) in a human weighing 70 kg (154 pounds). It is specialized to form hairs, nails, sweat, and oily glands (sebaceous). Skin is divided into the top layer (epidermis), the middle part (dermis), and the bottom layer (subdermis) or subcutaneous tissue (see the diagram). The epidermis has five layers of cells stacked one on top of another (Fig. 9):

1. Stratum corneum: 25-30 layers of cells filled with keratin, provides a water-proofing protection.
2. Stratum lucidum: several rows of clear cells containing eleidin, a precursor of keratin.

3. Stratum granulosum or malphigi: 3-5 rows of flat cells containing keratohyalin, a precursor of eleidin.
4. Stratum spinosum: 8-10 rows of polyhedral cells. This layer contain Langerhans cells which play a vital role in immune defense of the skin. It also contain keratinocytes described below.
5. Stratum basales: a single layer of columnar cells which divide and give rise to other cells in the epidermis. This layer also contain Merckel discs sensitive to touch.

The thickness of these cell layers varies from place to place. The epidermis has no blood vessels. It gets its nutrition through the blood vessels (capillaries) below the epidermis. Every day, thousands of skin cells are shed without our notice. It is estimated that during our 70-year life span, our bodies shed about 40 pounds of skin.

According to Dr. Irwin I. Lubowe, M.D., author of *New Hope for Your Skin*, published by E. P. Dutton & Company, Inc., (1962), each square inch of skin (all three layers) contains the following: 78 nerves, 650 sweat glands, 78 sensory apparatuses for heat, 13 sensory apparatuses for cold, 1,300 nerve endings to record pain, 19,500 sensory cells at the ends of nerve fibers, 165 pressure apparatuses for sense of touch and pressure, 100 sebaceous glands, 195,000,000 cells of different kinds. There are special kinds of cells in basal layer called Merkel cells involved in sensory function and/or adrenal gland-like function.

Nails and hair are the modification of the epidermis (skin). There are about 300,000 to 500,000 hairs on the human body, of which 100,000 are on the scalp which grows 0.012 inches a day and 5 inches a year. Beard grows 0.15 inches a day.

Color of the Skin

There are no structural differences in the skin of different races except for the color (pigment). The pigment is produced by special cells called melanocytes. There are about two million cells located in the deeper layers of the epidermis (basal layer). Ultraviolet rays from the sun or another source stimulate the production of an enzyme (called tyrosinase) in the cells of the epidermis, which converts the protein tyrosine into the dark melanin pigment. This melanin pigment is pushed to the surface of the skin and gives the skin a brown, black, white, or tanned color. Black people have more of this pigment compared to white people. This pigment is missing in albinism. Melanin pigment production is regulated by two hormones, one produced by the adrenal gland (cortisone) and the other by the pituitary gland (melanocyte-stimulating hormone or MSH). Black hair color is due to melanin pigment and gray hair lack this pigment. The melanin pigment protects the skin from the harmful effects of the ultraviolet radiation from the sun.

Skin as a Protective Barrier (Fig. 9)

The skin plays an important role in the proper functioning of the body. The skin acts as a protective barrier. It prevents bacteria and many noxious chemicals from entering the body. Fatty acids from the sweat, sebaceous glands, and amino acids of the skin (cysteine and keratin), mix with carbon dioxide excreted in the sweat, sebaceous glands, and hair follicles. This mixture forms an acid coating covering the entire skin. It wards off bacterial infection and prevents bacterial penetration of the body. Like the kidneys, skin helps in the excretion of products of our metabolism through sweat (one quart on cold days, two quarts on warm days). When kidney function is impaired, the sweat glands will increase their activity, and take over part of the waste disposal job. Sweat is 98-99% water and contains organic acids and minerals. The skin has its own manufacturing plant. Its chief product is two grams of sebum produced by the sebaceous glands every day. It keeps the skin moist and protects against the drying effect of the weather.

The skin is a barrier to many substances which try to enter the body. Chemicals such as ammoniated mercury, oil of wintergreen, turpentine, alcohol, dimethylsulfoxide (DMSO), acetone, xylene, and urine are absorbed through the skin. They are excreted in the urine. Skin has the selective ability to absorb a few specific substances. This quality of the skin is used by physicians to administer hormones and drugs.

Skin as Sense Organ (Fig. 9)

The skin is an important sense organ containing many nerve endings which relay the sensations of heat, cold, pressure, and pain to the brain (see the diagram). Deeper layers of the skin (epidermis) contain special cells called Merkel cells. These cells are similar to neurons and are probably involved in sensory function. They contain thick, dense granules in the cytoplasm which resemble the granules in adrenal medullary cells and the carotid body. I believe that these cells, along with Langerhans cells and keratinocytes, play an important role in healing, protein and hormone synthesis, and immune system stimulation.

Maintenance of Body Temperature

Skin plays an important role in dissipating heat. The human body generates a lot of energy in the form of heat. The skin dissipates 2,500 calories of heat daily. This is enough to heat as much as 25 quarts (six gallons) of water to the boiling point. When the body temperature falls, the blood vessels of the skin shrink to a small size, thereby shutting off the heat loss. During exercise (and hyperthermia), heat is generated. The blood vessels dilate and lose more heat than usual. Thus, the skin helps to maintain a 98.6°F body temperature. Below the epidermis is the network of blood vessels, nerve fibers, and the lymph channels which follow blood vessels. Blood vessels are directly connected without intervening capillaries (see Fig. 9). This is helpful in body temperature regulation. Skin breathes by taking in oxygen and eliminating carbon dioxide. The skin's respiratory function is stepped up when the lungs are damaged. This helps, to a small extent, in the elimination of carbon dioxide.

Methods of Inducing Skin Hyperthermia

Hyperthermia of the skin can be induced by immersing the body in a tub filled with water at temperature of 112° F. Maintain that temperature by constantly adding hot water slowly. Temperature of the water higher than this can result in skin burns. It can be achieved by staying in the dry sauna at high setting also.

Effect of Hyperthermia and Dry Sauna on the Skin

About 400 cc (33 ounces) of blood passes through the skin per minute in an average adult. In severe cold it can decrease as much as 50 cc per minute. When skin is heated as in hyperthermia to the maximum, the blood vessels dilate and blood flow increases as mush as 2-3 liters per minute. That is immersing the body in hot water of about 108 to 112° F can heat large volume of blood because, the blood comes in contact with the water and heats it. The hyperthermia can be induced by the hot water or dry sauna method because of this reason.

I strongly recommend this form of hyperthermia for HIV positive, AIDS, Kaposi sarcoma, leprosy and other skin afflictions. I believe that the expensive, dangerous and life threatening procedures such as extracorporeal method is not needed. The investigators who are using the hyperthermia method to cure AIDS should have tried these methods. During hyperthermia with AUT, the blood circulation increases many fold. Production of sweat increases. The activity Langerhans cells increases. They may be temporarily disabled due to intense heat. Antibody and healing factor production by Keratinocytes increases. Many disease-causing cells and microbe cells of Kaposi's sarcoma die. That is why Kaposi sarcoma melt away with hyperthermia and AUT. Those suffering from Kaposi should immediately start immersing their body in hot water tubs with a constant temperature of 112 °F.

Immune Defense Cells of the Skin (Fig. 9, 10)

The deeper layers of epidermis contain spidery looking cells called Langerhans cells, which are derived from bone marrow. These cells have processes much like the tentacles of an octopus, which touch with the neighboring Langerhans cell processes. They form a continuous network in the skin like a fish net. Some of these cells migrate from the skin to regional lymph nodes. They have Ia, Fc, and C3 surface receptors like macrophages of the immune defense system. The lymphocytes gather around these cells after an antigenic challenge. These cells are involved in the presentation of antigens to lymphocytes.

These cells are the body's most important link between the outside and inside world. When any foreign antigen touches the skin, these cells make contact with it, pluck the antigen and its molecular fingerprints, present it to various immune defense cells. The immune system cells and its products are summoned to the rescue. For example, Langerhans cells are responsible for identifying poison oak and ivy. They set in motion an immune response resulting in rash, itching, swelling, and pain (a skin contact allergic response). Dr. Margaret Kripke, Ph.D., professor of immunology at the University of Texas, M. D. Anderson Cancer Center, says that damage to these cells can weaken the powers of the immune system in the distant part of the immune system. It is important to protect them to safeguard the general health. These cells are very sensitive; even a mild sunburn or ultraviolet radiation exposure disables them for a week.

When urine is applied externally, these cells pick up antigen from permeating urine and present it to the regional lymphocytes and lymph nodes. From there it is picked up by the immune defense system, resulting in the production of antibodies against that antigen which is causing the disease.

By applying urine all over the body, as well as by drinking it, the entire immune system is presented with the antigen. Then the immune system is stimulated to the maximum extent to fight the disease. Some of the urine is also absorbed by the blood and lymph vessels of the skin. Thus the antigen material circulates all over the body and is presented to the immune defense system organs and cells. The external application of urine should continue all through one's life.

Amazing Keratinocytes of the Skin (Fig. 9)

Research on the skin is revealing more of its secrets. Skin is the largest organ of the body. Cells of the deeper layers of skin are called keratinocytes. Because of their capacity to synthesize keratin, they are very active and perform many functions:

1. They manufacture a cholesterol transporting protein called apoprotein-E. Thus, they play a role in the body's transport and breakdown of cholesterol.

2. They break down some cancer-causing agents and make them harmless.
3. They convert less active thyroid hormone into the most active form.
4. They produce interleukin-I and 6, which stimulate different parts of the immune defense system.
5. They produce white blood cell stimulating factor called granulocyte-macrophage colony stimulating factor (GM-CSF). This stimulates new immune cell growth. Early studies show that these factors can be used to enhance and amplify the cellular response of the immune defense cells (JAMA, 1988, vol. 260, p. 355).
6. They produce a hormone similar to the one produced by the thymus gland. It probably helps in the maturation of lymphocytes into fully-developed, aggressive disease fighters.
7. These cells may become the pathway to the healing of the entire body. Interlukin-I, one of the substances produced by keratinocytes, is being tested as an enhancer of wound healing.
8. There is a possibility of inserting genes into the artificially grown keratinocytes and then putting them back within the body to produce hormones (insulin, growth hormones, etc.) and enzymes (pancreas).
9. AIDS patients with Kaposi's sarcoma live twice as long as other patients. This skin cancer is probably part of the natural protective processes of the body, a form of immune response. That is why the hyperthermia and AUT will be effective in Kaposis sarcoma. Keratinocytes may be helpful in rebuilding the immune system in AIDS patients.
10. The latest study has demonstrated that the recombinant human epidermal growth factors made by Chiron Labs of Emmerville, California, enhances the skin regeneration and growth (*New Eng J Med*, 1989, 321, p.76-79, 111-112).

There will be more discoveries made on this growth factor and other hormone-like substances produced by the skin cells. Autoimmune urine therapy, along with the external application of urine, hyperthermia increases the activity of all these cells and can play an important role in the treatment of various local and general diseases, including AIDS.

External Application of Urine - How and When?

Application of urine on the skin is a very important part of autoimmune urine therapy (Matthew 6:17, Isaiah 1:16). Autoimmune urine therapy without the use of it on the skin is well-expressed in Isaiah 1:30, "For you will be like an oak whose leaf fades away or as a garden that has no water." Autoimmune urine therapy practiced without rubbing it on the skin is compared to a garden without water and an oak tree without leaves--desolate and barren.

Collect morning urine and drink most of it. Save enough to apply all over the body from head to toe. Soft plastic bristled brushes or a wash cloth can be used to rub the urine into the skin. Apply the urine, let it dry for awhile, and then reapply. Massage the body with urine 1 to 2 hours at a time. J. W. Armstrong and his followers advocate using seven-day-old urine. The urine is collected every day in seven different wide-mouthed bottles. Begin using the urine from the oldest bottles.

If a person is undergoing hyperthermia therapy, finish the therapy, wait till the sweating is stopped and then apply urine on the skin.

Changes in Stored Urine

Urine stored for seven days loses its golden yellow color. It becomes flocculent and darkened due to oxidation of its pigment (urobilinogen). After standing in a container, the flocculent material separates and settles to the bottom of the collecting jar. It contains proteins (nucleoprotein and mucoprotein) and some epithelial cells from the lining of the genitourinary tract. Uric acid precipitates from acid urine. Calcium phosphate, ammonium and magnesium phosphate, oxalate, and urate, precipitate in alkaline urine. Stored urine develops a pungent smell. Before using old urine for massaging the body, shake well, and warm to a tepid temperature. I cannot argue for or against using old urine on the skin. Old urine should not be taken orally (drinking), injected, or applied to the eyes, nose, or ears, or used to gargle.

Allantoin in Urine

J. W. Armstrong, based on the communication he received from Dr. George G. Cotton of Temple, Texas, U.S.A., stated that the urine's external healing power was due to allantoin. The adult urine without allantoin has the healing power. Allantoin ($C4H6N4O3$) is found in allantoic fluid (fluid covering the fetus). It is a product of purine metabolism. It is found in most mammal's urine, but it is absent in humans and higher apes (chimpanzees, gorillas, orangutans). It is produced synthetically by oxidation of uric acid. It is possible that seven-day-old stored urine may contain allantoin due to oxidation of uric acid. That is probably one of the reasons old urine is much more effective on skin conditions, especially chronic ulcers, eczema, etc. Allantoin is used to encourage healing of chronic wounds, ulcers, and osteomyelitis. It is an active substance in maggot treatment. It is secreted by maggots as a product of purine metabolism. The healing power of urine is due to various organic and inorganic chemicals, enzymes, hormones, antigens, antibodies, pigments, urea, etc., contents of urine (JAMA 1979, vol. 241, pp. 1559-1563).

Urine for Aging Skin

Aging skin is a constant worry of Western men and women. There are two kinds of aging: (1) intrinsic aging and (2) photo-aging. Intrinsic aging refers to those skin changes due to internal (endogenous) factors. These are unknown and may be due to genetically-programmed aging (senescence). The skin in these conditions shows thinning (epidermoid atrophy), loss of elasticity, deepening of normal expression lines--so-called wrinkles (retraction of retae pegs, dermal atrophy, flattening of dermo epithelial interface). On the other hand, photo aging (dermato-heliosis) is characterized by wrinkles, yellow lax rough leathery blood shot skin with hypo- or hyperpigmented spots (epidermal dysplasia, loss of polarity of keratinocytes, dermal damage with marked elastosis, loss of collagen, increased glycosamnioglycans, infiltration of inflammatory white blood cells).

The sun's ultra violet rays causes this kind of damage. This condition of photo-aging is preventable by use of sun-screens and avoidance of ultraviolet light and sunlight. These conditions of skin aging may not be preventable completely. It is delayed by application of urine on the body, especially on the hands, face, and neck (areas exposed to the sun). Photo-aging is preventable and reversible to some extent. Recent experiments with application of 0.1% Tretinion Cream (Retin A - ointment, Ortho Pharmaceutical Corp.) a Vitamin A derivative, can reverse the photo-aging (JAMA, 1988, vol. 259, p. 527). Consult with your physician to obtain a prescription to use it. It is expensive.

The cheapest prescription-free drug, we have is application of urine. Urine is applied to the skin. Include the skin exposed to the sunlight, such as hands, face, and neck (back and front). Urine acts on the epidermis by helping cell differentiation, peptide growth factor modulation, cell division, RNA and protein synthesis, post-transnational glycorylation of proteins, and prostaglandin biosynthesis. It is an excellent antiseptic. There is no adverse reaction to the application of urine (old or new). There are adverse reactions to application of Retin-A Ointment. It can change the color of the skin to pink and cause dermatitis, and inflammation (subclinical actinic keratosis).

One of the best skin lotions produced by a multi-billion dollar drug company contains 10% urea. This cream maintains skin moisture and smoothness longer than any other cream I have tested. I see many old patients with horrible skin conditions (dry, scaly, infected, rough, broken, wrinkled, blistered, hemorrhagic patches, infected hair follicles) in our hospital. They can be helped by the application of urine in the home and at the hospitals. They will be completely free of all skin afflictions and look fine. My wife uses morning urine on her face and applies light make-up over it. It is an excellent base for make-up application. Kaposis and some skin conditions can be helped by hyperthermia and AUT. Hyperthermia may not be useful for all the skin conditions.

Urine Application for Skin Conditions (burns, open wounds , eczema, lupus, psoriasis, keratitis, athletes foot, dandruff, herpes, herpes zoster, Kaposi sarcoma, and skin lesions in AIDS, etc.)

Though the application of old urine externally is helpful, only fresh urine should be used for oral use (drinking). Old urine is used on old dry lesions of the skin such as psoriasis, lupus, eczema, skin lesions of leprosy, dry gangrene, keratitis, dandruff, scruff, papillomas, athlete's foot, various fungus infections, allergic dermatitis, poison ivy, Kaposi's sarcoma, and various skin conditions associated with AIDS, etc. Fresh urine is applied for fresh wounds such as cuts, burns, allergic lesions, and stings. If the lesion is chronic, meaning many weeks old, and refuses to heal, use urine-soaked packs and keep the lesion wet by applying urine repeatedly. I use a bottle with an air pump spray. It is filled with urine and sprayed on the lesion. Urine can be safely applied on all skin lesions, new and old.

Many dermatologists recommend steroids containing ointments for various skin allergic conditions. These ointments are sold over the counter. The public is using them in large quantities. There is no ointment containing steroids which is as good and effective as urine application. Besides, urine costs nothing. Urine application outside the body should accompany total autoimmune urine therapy, lasting 1 to 24 weeks, depending on the condition. This is a must for extensive skin conditions covering wide areas of skin and for a chronic condition. I saw an old lady suffering from the herpes of the chest wall with severe pain. She got total relief of pain and healing of herpes lesions with external application of her own urine 4 to 6 times a day in less than a week. Pain was gone the same day.

Use of Urea on Surgical Wounds and Bad Nails (experiences in Russia and America)

Eugene M. Farber, M.D., and David A. South, M.D., Stanford University dermatologists, reported (JAMA, 1979, vol. 241, no. 15, pp. 1559-1563) the use of urea plasters for removing traumatized, diseased (dystrophic) nails instead of surgery. This method is used in the Soviet Union as a standard method. Surgery involves anesthesia, sepsis, and post-operative pain and exorbitant expense. This procedure is painless and less expensive. There is no risk of infection and bleeding compared with the surgical procedure. These dermatologists removed 116 toenails and 39 fingernails by the urea plaster method. They used a combination of urea, anhydrous, lanolin, white wax, and white petroleum. The nails had onychomalacia, psoriasis, bacterial infection, traumatic injury, and structural nail dystrophies.

After cleaning the affected nails with tincture of benzoin, the urea compound was applied to the affected nail surface, covered with a piece of plastic wrap, and covered with an adhesive tape or a finger cut out from a plastic glove. Patients were told to keep the area completely dry for ten days. Within five to ten days, most of the diseased nails were ready to be removed by macerating them. The normal nails were left intact. Most of these patients suffered no pain or infection. They might develop contact dermatitis when the tape was used to cover the area and occasional pinpoint bleeding when the diseased nail was removed. The lesions healed without any treatment. Not a single patient developed infection, which is not uncommon after surgical removal of the diseased nail.

Drs. Farber and South ascribe many properties to urea, such as antibacterial (kills bacterial causing disease), antifungal, antipruritic (prevents itching), keratolytic (removes dead skin dander, nails, and hair), protein solvent (dissolves and disintegrates the dead protein molecules), and it is a dehydrating agent (absorbs the water and edematous fluids from the surrounding area). They attribute wound-healing properties of urea for its excellent skin penetration. According to Drs. Farber and South, "Its most outstanding characteristics are that it is neither toxic nor allergic." It is also inexpensive. Dr. Wallace McLeod of the Georgia Baptist Medical Center Skin Department uses this urea preparation with excellent results.

Skin Cancers

There is bad news for sun worshippers, according to the American Cancer Society. Malignant melanoma, arising from a nevus or mole (dark, black, or brown spots on the skin), has increased by 93% in the last eight years. Skin cancer (basal cell carcinoma) are less malignant It affects three out of ten adults in the USA. Now four out of ten people born after 1985 develop it. At present, it affects 5,000,000 people in the United States. That figure could double in 25 years. The reason for this increase is due to heavy tanning in the 1950's and 1960's. It takes almost 20 years after heavy exposure to ultraviolet rays to develop skin cancer.

There are about 22,000 tanning salons in the United States and they are increasing at a 16% rate yearly. Tanning booths deliver four times more ultraviolet A radiation than sun rays. The ozone layer which protects us from damaging ultraviolet rays from the sun is becoming depleted. At the current rate, 40% of the ozone layer will be gone by the year 2075. This is exposing us to higher doses of the sun's UV rays. This will cause additional skin cancer in 154 million people in the world. An estimated 3.2 million will die from it. Applying urine before tanning will minimize the damage. Use sun screens to prevent the penetration of UV rays into the skin layers. Do not expose yourself more than 20 minutes at a time. If you use a sun cover like No. 15, you can stay up to 5 hours in the sun (15 x 20 = 300 minutes) with the same effect. By multiplying 20 by the sun screen factor (SSF), this gives the number of minutes a person can stay in the sun for tanning purposes.

Kaposi's sarcoma is a cancer of the skin, as well as other internal organs, seen in immune deficiency syndromes, including AIDS. Rubbing urine on skin lesions and then applying urine soaked liniments 3 to 4 times a day along with total autoimmune urine therapy along with skin hyperthermia has a good chance of healing this condition. This also reduces the chances of opportunistic infection which kills these patients (discussed in detail in Chapter 18).

Urine for Hair Growth and Dandruff

There are reported cases of hair growing back and even becoming dark in color after applying urine on the scalp. Many people reported decline or stoppage of hair loss after applying urine on the scalp. The same phenomenon was noticed by myself. My hair became so thick my sister-in-law asked whether I was wearing artificial hair. I told her to pass her fingers through my hair and feel for herself. This is far better and less expensive than minoxidil (Rogain) marketed as a hair-growing miracle drug. This anti-hypertensive drug makes the hair grow. These new hairs are thin and fuzzy, and will disappear if the use of the drug is discontinued.

Urine, along with its various contents, including urea, opens up blocked hair follicles. It clears away all of the dandruff, make the scalp healthier and stimulate the hair growth. The hair loss stops or brought under control. The scalp should be covered with a plastic cap so the urine will not evaporate easily. The urine is applied repeatedly all day and then the scalp is washed with tepid water. If needed, use a mild shampoo. This is the best, cost-free drug available for hair loss. Urine is an excellent keratolytic, meaning it clears away all dandruff of the scalp and inhibits dandruff formation. I have used it with excellent results on my scalp to clear dandruff and prevent hair loss.

Eczema and Dermatitis

The terms dermatitis and eczema are almost synonymous. They refer to inflammation of the skin of an allergic nature. This is the response of the skin to a variety of agents such as bacteria, viruses, fungus, proteins, and contact with poisonous plants (poison ivy), etc. The allergen which causes this condition can act from outside or inside the body. This eczematous condition can be either acute, subacute, or chronic.

There are many kinds of eczematous conditions such as contact dermatitis, nummular eczema, atopic dermatitis, lichen simplex chronicus, exudative discoid and lichenoid chronic dermatosis, seborrheic dermatitis, stasis dermatitis, generalized exfoliative dermatitis, etc. AIDS patients suffer from many kinds of dermatitis and eczematous lesions also. Wash these lesions and apply urine three to six times a day. If the lesion has been existing for a long time, apply new or old urine soaked liniments on it. It may be helpful to practice skin hyperthermia as described above and in Chapter 1. This therapy will help to augment the healing processes. All it needs is immersing the limb in hot water at 112°F. for 3-4 hours. External urine application, followed by total autoimmune urine therapy, is also recommended for a week or two.

Autoimmune urine therapy is very effective in all kinds of skin conditions. I would try it before any other treatment. When urine is applied on the skin to eczematous and skin allergic conditions, the antigens causing this conditions penetrate the skin. The urine helps the penetration of these substances into the deeper layer of the skin. The Langerhans cells and keratinocytes of the skin pick up these allergens and causative agents. They present them to the immune defense system which produce antibodies to act against the allergens and disease. Keratinocytes are stimulated to enhance the immune system.

Applying urine every day is like getting desensitization shots for various allergic conditions. Urine kills all the bacteria which are growing on the skin. It neutralizes the irritants that are found in the toxic plants (poison ivy) and chemicals. It is a sure remedy for poison ivy and insect stings. It enhances the healing processes in skin burns. In general, it is an excellent enhancer of the healing process of the skin. Hyperthermia enhances the activity of Langerhans cells and keratinocytes. It also kills the bacteria, the cells about to become cancer(precancerous cells) and cancer cells in the skin.

Urine application after hyperthermia enhances the healing processes. Because more urine is absorbed from the skin due to increased circulation and loosening of the skin layers and between skin cells.

FIGURE 9: SHOWING THE COMPLICATED STRUCTURE OF THE SKIN. EPIDERMIS HAS NO BLOOD VESSELS. NERVES, BLOOD VESSELS, HAIR ROOTS, SKIN GLANDS, FAT, ETC. ARE LOCATED BELOW THE EPIDERMIS.

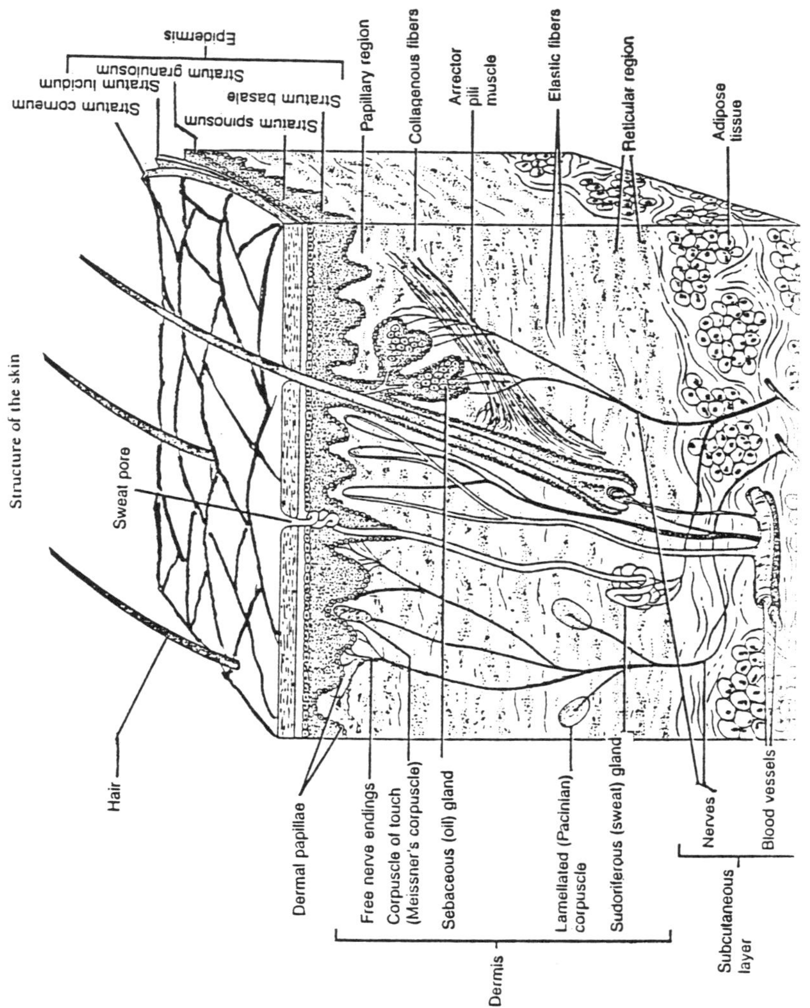

FIGURE 10: SHOWS LANGERHANS IMMUNE DEFENSE CELLS LOCATED IN THE SKIN. THEY HAVE PROCESSES LIKE OCTOPUS SPREAD ON THE SKIN LIKE A FISH NET AND PICK UP ANTIGENS FROM SKIN.

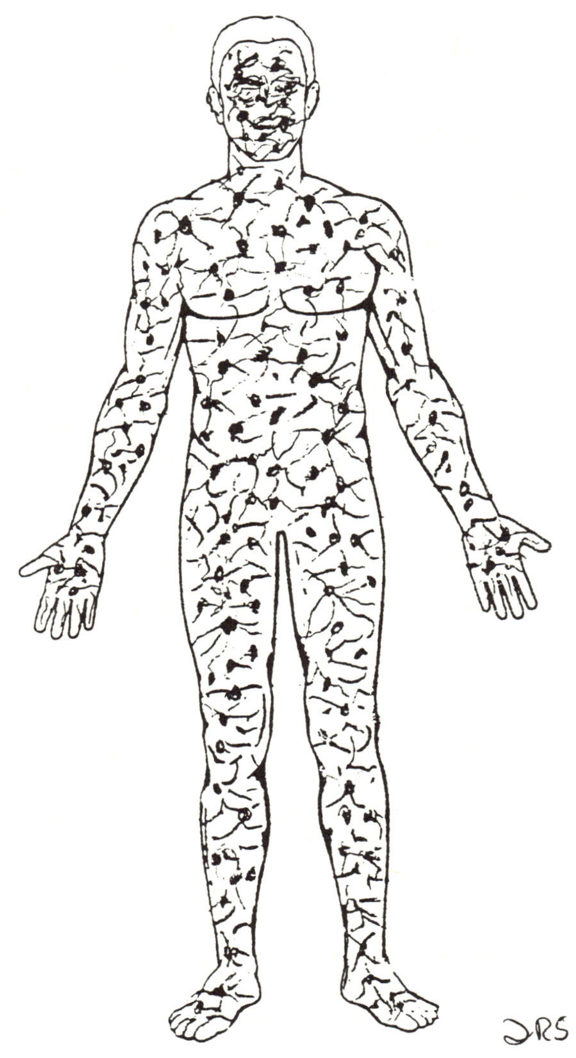

CHAPTER 15

ACQUIRED IMMUNE DEFICIENCY SYNDROME (AIDS)

I am the one who has the body,
You are the one who has the breath.
You know the secrets of my body,
I know the secret of your breath.
That is why your body is mine,
Your breath in my body.
Oh God Ramanatha (Shiva).

Devara Dasimayya
12th Century Shiva Saint from India

Nothing is more terrible than ignorance in action.

Goethe

Background

AIDS is the acronym for acquired immune deficiency syndrome. Acquired means the disease is passed from one person to another and is not inherited. The immune system defending the body is affected. There is a deficiency in the immune defense mechanism. Syndrome means a group of symptoms occurring together. There are thousands of articles and hundreds of books written on this subject. This disease is a plague of the 20th Century. It has already claimed more than 90,000 lives (by 1990) in the United States and 300,000 lives all around the world. AIDS cases are showing up in most countries. Millions (1-1/2 to 2 million in the U.S. alone) of people are harboring the AIDS virus (HIV seropositive). Many of these people will develop the full-blown disease within eight years.

This disease as an entity was not recognized for a long time. In June, 1981 the Centers for Disease Control of Atlanta published a report of the unusual occurrence of five cases of pneumocystis carinii (a protozoa) pneumonia (PCP) among five healthy homosexuals. This was followed with reports of Kaposi sarcoma (a skin cancer) occurring in young gay men. Soon more reports began to follow. PCP had been observed previously only in severe immuno-suppressed patients. Soon, with hundreds of these cases, the title AIDS was given.

About 75% of the people who contact AIDS will die five years following diagnosis. With advances in treatment survival time is increasing. AIDS has been linked to a wide range of lethal opportunistic infections and unusual tumors (see Chapter 16). The initial appearance of AIDS among homosexuals prompted speculations that the lifestyle gay men lead with chronic cytomegalovirus exposure to coexisting sexually transmitted disease and the use of recreational drugs (amyl nitrate, speed, cocaine, marijuana, heroin, narcotics, etc.) was blamed as the possible causative factor for the immune suppression seen in AIDS.

Isolating the AIDS Virus (Fig. 11)

By 1981, AIDS was reported among heterosexuals and intravenous drug abusers. Five cases of AIDS were reported among hemophiliacs followed by reports of AIDS development after blood transfusions. These reports led investigators to believe that AIDS is caused by an infectious agent transmitted through the blood and its products. In 1983, L. Montagnier at the Pasteur Institute in Paris, and early in 1984 Robert Gallo at the National Cancer Institute in the United States, isolated the virus from AIDS patients. The virus was named lymphadenopathy virus (LAV) or human T cell lymphotrophic virus Type III (HTLV-III), respectively. These viruses were also called AIDS-associated retrovirus (ARV). Currently, human immune deficiency virus (HIV) is the internationally accepted nomenclature. The AIDS virus is a retrovirus, indicating that these viruses carry their genetic material in RNA rather than DNA. Dr. Robert C.

Gallo, has contributed immensely in understanding HIV and other related retroviruses (Scientific American, December, 1986, no. 6, p. 255, and January, 1987, no. 1, p. 256).

Live AIDS virus has been isolated from blood, semen, urine, vaginal secretions, bone marrow, lymph nodes, spleen, cerebrospinal fluid, brain and neural tissue, tears, breast milk and saliva, chromaffin cells of the rectum, duodenum, colon tissue, dendritic cells in the skin, mucous membranes, lymph nodes, liver, spleen and brain.

The immune defect seen in this disease was traced to a specific subset of T lymphocytes, the helper/inducer T4 cells. This retrovirus attacks this group of lymphocytes and kills them. It is interesting to note that the antibody to HIV does not appear to be protective. On the contrary it is often a reliable marker of the presence of the live infective virus. For every 50 to 100 people infected with the AIDS virus, there is one case of AIDS.

Plagues of the World

The world has faced plagues throughout the history of mankind. The black death (plague) between 1347 and 1350 killed almost 25 to 50% of the European population (25 to 50 million). It killed more people in less time than any other disease. The plague came under control only when the population who were sick developed an increasing immunity and recovered.

Smallpox killed more than 400,000 people in Europe during the 18th Century. It did not discriminate between common man and royalty. The Queen of Sweden also succumbed to this disease in 1741.

Between 1917 and 1918 an estimated 22 million people died from a worldwide outbreak of influenza. Influenza killed half the people in my own family. My father had an attack and recovered from the disease. Louse-born typhus devastated the Russian and Polish population. Three million people died between 1917 and 1922 before the disease ran its course. More than 400,000 Americans were infected with polio between 1943 and 1956 and killed 22,000 by paralysis and respiratory failure. After the introduction of the Salk

(1955) and Sabin (1961) vaccines, polio has almost completely disappeared.

AIDS: A 20th Century Plague

The first verifiable case of AIDS in the United States is that of a 15-year-old boy. He died of immune depression in 1968. His organs and blood were cold preserved, and recent tests have shown that his blood serum is positive for AIDS. Lancet in july 7th. 1990 issue reported a case of AIDS from the preserved tissues of a dead sailor stored for 31 years. This sailor died of mysterious viral disease in 1959. This if is the first recorded case of AIDS. I think that the AIDS was around even before 1950's but was not recognized. The AIDS epidemic began over ten years later. Federal health officials project that 365,000 Americans will develop AIDS by the end of 1992. It may strike 100,000 new people during that year. Since 1981, 120,000 Americans have developed AIDS and 90,000 have died. By 1991, between 10,000 and 20,000 infants and children will be infected with the AIDS virus. By the end of 1991, the AIDS death toll will reach 270,000, and 450,000 will die by 1993. Out of 5 million U.S. military men tested, 6,000 were tested HIV positive. In another study 1 in 500 U.S. university students were positive. An estimated 1.5 to 2 million Americans are said to be HIV positive.

We cannot compare AIDS to the other plagues, because AIDS is difficult to contract. Unlike the black death, insect bites play no role in its spread, and AIDS is not spread by mosquito bites. One important aspect of AIDS, compared to other previous plagues is that AIDS is always lethal. It is transmitted by the most basic human action called sex. For just that reason, the AIDS virus will cause a "sexual revolution" as the birth control pill did in the sixties. Sexual promiscuity and multiple sexual partners may become a thing of the past. People who value their life may even ask their would-be partners to undergo a blood test before engaging in a sexual relationship or marriage. The password is "practice safe sex." Have sex with partners whom you know well, if uncertain, use a condom.

What Are Viruses?

Virus in Latin means slimy liquid or poison. Viruses are smaller than a millionth of an inch in diameter. They can be seen only under the electron microscope. They cannot be seen with the ordinary microscope used in a doctor's office. They are the biologic ultimate of a parasite. They cannot exist on their own and need a living host cell to multiply and propagate. Viruses are specks of protein enclosed in an envelop of fat, carbohydrate and complex. They cause almost 75 to 80% of all acute illnesses in the United States, such as influenza and the common cold. They also cause fatal diseases such as rabies, small pox, yellow fever, and polio, as well as the 20th Century plague, AIDS. Scientists are beginning to suspect that the virus may play an important role in heart disease, birth defects, diabetes, Alzheimer's disease, cancers, multiple sclerosis, etc., twenty out of sixty multiple sclerosis patients showed a virus in their brain fluid (CSF) according to a report from Baylor College of Medicine in Houston. There are 250,000 Americans who suffer from this disease. Another member of the AIDS causing virus called HTLV-I as well as it cousin HTLV-II cause a rare form of leukemia in humans.

Viruses Cannot Exist on Their Own and Need Our Body to Reproduce and Survive

Viruses cannot reproduce on their own and cannot perform basic functions as other living cells do. They must invade living cells in plants, animals or humans where they command the cell's genetic material to multiply and produce new viruses. They are totally dependent on living cells. The living cells in our body are made up of very complex chemicals. They are capable of independent existence. They produce many proteins, grow, multiply, extract energy from food, and react to changes in their environment. Viruses do not have many of these capacities. The type of disease they cause depends on the type of cell and the organ they invade. For example, influenza viruses attack the respiratory tract, the AIDS virus attacks T4 lymphocytes of the immune system, the polio virus attacks the spinal cord nerve cells, rabies attacks the brain cells, the hepatitis virus attacks the liver, etc.

Why do Viruses Attack a Specific System Cells in Our Body?

The reason viruses attack a particular type of cell is explained on the basis of receptors on the host cells. The proteins on the virus coating gets attracted and attached to these receptors. There are different kinds of proteins which envelop the virus and the genetic material. The function of one such protein is to attach to the cell receptor. Another one weakens the cell membrane so the virus can get into the cell. A third one changes the cell to produce viral progeny and so on.

Newly-formed viruses from inside the host cell are released by a process called budding. The newly-formed virus pushes out through the cell membrane. This bubble-like bulge breaks away from the cell. The newly-released virus floats away to infect new cells. The wounded cells are impaired or unable to repair its damaged cell membrane. The contents of the cell leak, collapsing it like a punctured balloon, and the cell dies.

Many of these microbes, after initial attack, escape the immune mechanism and hide. They cause disease later when resistance (immunity) falls. The classic example is the chicken pox virus. It can cause painful shingles years after it has triggered the mild childhood disease. The hepatitis B virus causes liver cancer. The papilloma virus causes genital warts and later can cause cervical cancer in women. There are many indications that hidden viruses are responsible for many cancers, especially leukemia. Now there is evidence that the AIDS virus may be hiding in the red bone marrow cells which produce various cells in the blood. There is a good possibility that some of these viruses and virus infected cells get flushed out during hyperthermia and AUT.

Origin of the AIDS Virus

Where did this deadly AIDS virus come from? Is it a product of natural mutation or evolution from another virus or is it sent by God? The first member of the HTLV family, HTLV-1, is endemic in parts of Africa, Caribbean Islands, Southeastern United States, South America and Japan. In 1978, HTLV-1 was implicated in T cell cancers in humans. This virus is related to Simian T lymphotrophic virus type-1 (STLV-1) found in Old World monkeys (green monkey in Africa). HTLV-1 represents a variation of Simian virus emerged from a common ancestor in Africa. HTLV-1 was spread through commercial and slave trading routes dating back to the 16th century. Another virus similar to HIV causes AIDS in the macaques only. These findings show that HTLV-III (HIV) emerged from Africa through genetic variation among pre-existing entities. There is also molecular and biologic evidence that HTLV-III may be related to the Lenti virus family which cause progressive debilitating diseases in hoofed animals. The HTLV-I, II, III are interrelated and causes different human diseases. It is definitely not God sent, man made or Russian plot.

AIDS Virus Appearance and Its Genes (Fig. 11)

At present, the U.S. government spends billions of dollars annually on AIDS research and education. Scientists have developed a pretty good sketch of the AIDS virus. By using various scientific tools, including the electron microscope, researchers know how it looks. It looks like a golf ball which has a dimpled surface covered with glycoprotein buttons. They have mapped the genetic code and know where the individual genes lie and what role they play in directing the activity of the virus. This is the most investigated virus in the history of virology. Researchers even have discovered a segment of human genetic material called Kappa B on the HIV genetic structure. This discovery has prompted the speculation that years ago, the virus hijacked part of a gene from the human host, a mutation that may have helped convert a harmless germ into a killer. This Kappa B gene acts as a switch which stimulates viral reproduction. The role of the Kappa B gene in the human cell is not known.

T4 lymphocyte have on its surface a receptor protein called CD4 which makes it possible for the immune system to identify alien invaders. It also exerts an irresistible attraction for a glycoprotein (GP-120) on the surface of the AIDS virus. It is like a magnet attracting bits of iron. Once it attaches to CD4 molecules, the virus begins to enter the T4 lymphocyte. If we can prevent the virus attaching to T4 receptors, we may have the solution to AIDS. I do believe that autoimmune urine therapy alters the mutual attraction to such a level as to prevent the HIV attachment to the T4 cells.

The work of many virologists such as W. Hazeltine, M. Essex, F. W. Staal at Harvard and NCI has shown that the AIDS virus has nine genes.

HIV Genes and Their Functions (Fig. 11):

1. GA: Coding for viral core proteins
2. POL: Specific for reverse transcriptase enzymes
3. ENV: External envelope protein
4. REV (ART, TRS): Differential regulator
5. VIF (R, A, P, Q): May produce antigen infectivity factor
6. TAT (TAT-3, TA): Positive regulator
7. VPR (R): Function not known
8. VPU: Function not known
9. NEF (3'ORF, B, E'F): Negative regulator

HIV is a retrovirus, meaning that the genetic material is in a single strand of RNA instead of the double helix of the DNA viruses. Once inside the T4 lymphocytes, the virus, with the help of an enzyme reverse transcriptase, directs HIV into a double stranded DNA gene. It then incorporates these copies into genes (DNA) of the host cells. Azidothymidine (AZT), used to treat AIDS victims, inhibits the production of reverse transcriptase. Though AZT does not cure the disease, it interferes with the ability to spread by forming DNA. To be effective against AIDS, the drug should act on the virus, as well as the infected cells. The inside of the infected T4 cell becomes a viral factory. The viral material gathers under the cell surface membrane. This gradually organizes into a virion. It pinches off from the cell's outer surface moves into circulation and attacks new T4 lymphocytes.

Immune System Involved in AIDS (Fig. 12)

Let us examine what happens in AIDS. We have already described how the immune defense system works in the body in a previous chapter. We will recount it here briefly. The mother cells (pluripotential stem cells) of the red bone marrow give rise to several kinds of white blood cells such as granulocyte, lymphocytes and monocytes and macrophages, as well as to red blood cells (which carry oxygen) and platelets (which participate in blood clotting).

Lymphocytes are further divided into B and T cells. B cells mature in the bone marrow when stimulated by an antigen and give rise to memory B cells and antibody secreting plasma cells. The memory B cells retain the ability to recognize specific antigen long after initial exposure has disappeared and divides, giving rise to millions of B cells and antibody secreting plasma cells. These antibodies attack the antigen thus contributing to long-term immunity (humoral immunity). AUT and hyperthermia enhances the activity of T and B cells and increases their output of humoral substances and antibodies.

T Cells (Fig.6, 7)

T cells develop in the thymus gland (located behind the breast bone) and are distributed all over the body and in the blood. Sixty to seventy percent of the lymphocytes in the circulating blood are T cells. They are further divided into:

1. Cytotoxic T cells which attack and kill foreign cells and infected cells.
2. Helper T cells which recognize foreign antigen and help activate cytotoxic T cells and antibody-producing B cells.
3. Inducer T cells which help to promote the different subsets of T cells.
4. Suppressor T cells which help suppress the response of other cells. These cells help to provide a feedback regulation system, so the other three types of T cells do not overdo their job.

T cells are also classified structurally by their surface receptors:

1. Those which display T4 antigen receptors comprise the helper/inducer cells.
2. Those which show T8 antigen are comprised of cytotoxic/suppressor T cells.

Function of T Cells and Macrophages (Fig. 6, 12)

In response to antigen (infection) the macrophages first engulf the pathogen and produce a secretion called Interleukin-I. This Interleukin-I and antigen further stimulate all types of lymphocytes (T and B cells). T cell stimulation causes production of a protein lymphokine called Interleukin-II which activates the B cell system. T4 cells produce alpha interferon which stimulates macrophages and natural killer T cells. Thus the T4 cells help amplify the response of other immune system cells many times to fight the infection. These activated macrophages, natural killer cells, cytotoxic T cells, and antibody-producing plasma cells help to provide an effective immune defense against invading antigens (virus, bacteria, cancer cells, foreign cells, etc.).

T4 cells, like an orchestra conductor, play a pivotal role in the overall modulation of this immune response by producing Interlukin-II and alpha interferon, recognizing foreign antigens, causing clonal cell proliferation of T cells, mediating suppressor/cytotoxic functions and helping B cells to produce a specific antibody. Now we can understand what a devastating affect it will have on the immune defense system if the T4 lymphocytes are depleted.

All the infectious complications (opportunistic infections) of AIDS are explained on the basis of the HIV virus infection of T4 cells and their ultimate demise due to the killing (cytopathic) action of HIV on T4 cells. There is a reduced number of T4 cells (lymphopenia), which increases the susceptibility to a wide range of opportunistic infections and neoplasms (tumors, Kaposi sarcoma). The normal ratio of T4 to T8 cells is higher than 1.00. In AIDS patients it is lower than 0.5. Healthy blood contain 1000 to 2000 T4 cells per cubic milliliter of blood. In AIDS patients it is between a few cells to 400 per cubic milliliter of blood. AUT and hyperthermia increases the T4 cells and reverses the ratio. There is a good possibility that T4 cells and antibody level goes up in blood within ten days of therapy.

Immune Regulation Disruption (Fig. 6, 12)

A normal immune response depends on fairly precise and complex interactions between many different elements. The reduction of T4 cell subsets disrupts this coordinated precise response. Even delayed hypersensitivity of the skin is reduced or absent. The clones of T and B cells do not proliferate with the same vigor. Activity of all other subsets of T cells is inhibited. Due to the diminished recognition of antigen and decreased T4 cell production of Interleukin-II, macrophages show decreased chemotaxis, cell killing affect, and diminished production of Interlukin-I. B cells (plasma cells) respond poorly to antigen stimulation and produce a smaller amount of poor quality antibody. That is why there is elevated immunoglobulin associated with impaired human immunity.

In AIDS there is defect in cellular elements, lymphokine production, and antibody synthesis. Many immune system suppressor factors are produced in AIDS. As the AIDS virus attacks T4 cells, this disease can be easily called a disease associated with immunoregulation rather than immunosuppression (see the diagrams). AUT and hyperthermia eliminates or diminishes the effects of immune system suppressor factors.

How HIV Attacks T4 Lymphocytes (Fig. 12, 13)

To gain contact with these lymphocytes, the AIDS virus needs access to the blood circulation of the host. The virus gets into the host due to breakdown in the mucous membrane of the anus and rectum and other sexual organs, blood transfusions, needle sticks and body secretions. Once the virus is in the circulation, the surface protein (CD4) of the T4 cells acts as a receptor site for the AIDS virus.

After the virus attaches to T4 cell receptors, it is drawn into the cell by creating a hole in the cell wall. The HIV can enter brain cells and fibroblasts in vitro. Studies show other cell surface receptor sites are involved in AIDS virus attachment and entry into the cells. The HIV surface contains gp 41. It is made up of a nucleotide sequence resembling fusion-inducing regions of Paramyxo viruses. So it is likely that the HIV gp 120 attaches to the cell's CD4 receptors. Fusion of the HIV gp 41 domain with the cell membrane is needed for bringing the viral core inside the host cell (JAMA 1989, vol. 261, pp. 2997-3006). AUT and hyperthermia prevents attachment of AIDS Virus and its entrance into the susceptible cells such as T4 cells by altering the gp 41 domain of the HIV.

The most important discovery made in virology was finding the reverse transcriptase enzyme. It helps the RNA virus produce a copy of DNA with the same code. Without such conversion, RNA viruses reach a dead end street inside the cell. Howard M. Temin and David Baltimore were awarded the Nobel Prize in Medicine for their 1970 discovery ("RNA Directed DNA Synthesis," by Howard T. Temin, Scientific American, January, 1972).

HIV Viral Multiplication and Killing of T4 Cells (Fig. 13)

The virus inside the T4 lymphocyte may remain dormant for years until stimulated. That is why the incubation period for the virus is so variable, from weeks to years. Why the virus multiples when the T4 cells multiply is not known. The DNA sequences for Lymphokine Interlukin-II and alpha interferon are the same as for the provirus in the T4 cell. When the T4 cell is stimulated by antigen to produce Interlukin-II, alpha interferon and T4 cell division, this hidden provirus also divides. That means the same immunologic signal could activate both AID virus multiplication and lymphokines production processes through their related genetic pathway. This virus bursts into such a fury of activity inside the cell that they fill the lymphocyte. They make holes on the cell membrane as they emerge out of the T4 cells. This results in leakage of important parts of cytoplasm like a punctured balloon, leading to death. This action is called the cytopathic action of the virus.

The speed and efficiency of viral replication is aided by the gene in the virus (transacting transcriptional activation). This gene helps the transcription of viral RNA into protein. The viral particles released from the dead or dying T4 cell attack other T4 cells. After a critical point, depletion of the T cell begins, resulting in the clinical manifestation of AIDS.

The HIV viruses do kill the T4 cells, but it is not enough for such massive depletion seen in AID patients. According to Dr. Robert Gallo of NCI, the T4 cell depletion can also be due to:

1. Fusion of infected T4 cells with uninfected cells (syncytia).
2. The result of an auto immune response.
3. As HIV particles leave the host cell, a molecule called gp-120 falls off the outer viral coat. This can bind to CD4 molecule of

uninfected cell. Such T4 lymphocytes get marked and destroyed by immune system.

4. When HIV binds to T4 cells, an enzyme called protease is released. This enzyme digests proteins. Large quantities of this enzyme released during a viral attack might weaken white blood cells and shorten their lives.

AUT and hyperthermia reverses some of these processes and increases T4 cell content by reducing their destruction.

Why Do T4 Cells Die and Other Cells Survive? (Fig. 13)

The number of CD_4 molecules on macrophages and monocytes are considerably less compared to T4 lymphocytes. The rate of killing of the cells is directly proportional to the number of CD_4 receptors. More of the CD_4 receptors found on a cell, more chances of death due to HIV infection. Monocytes and macrophages have fewer CD_4 receptors and do not die easily. Another explanation is that the death of a cell depends upon the interaction between the viral envelop and the host cell membrane. As the virus buds out, holes are created in the host cell membrane. If the holes can be repaired fast enough, the cell will not die. If they are not closed as fast as they are made, the vital cell contents leak out and the cells die. It is possible that CD_4 receptors carrying monocytes and macrophages repair the cell wall rapidly, allowing the cell to survive. As there are fewer numbers of CD_4 receptors in these cells, fewer number of liberated proviruses bud off. This results in fewer holes on the cell membrane which are easily repaired

Infected T4 cells, when activated, yield only ten T4 cells instead of the 1,000 progeny normally seen. Besides depletion of T4 cells, there is a drastic reduction in memory clones on the T4 cells. This factor also plays a major role in AIDS. Why only the T4 lymphocytes is affected is explained by the following novel experiment. When the T4 gene is inserted into a cell which does not carry the infection due to lack of CD_4 surface marker, the viral infection is acquired. Therefore, the CD_4 surface marker is important for this virus to attack. The CD4 surface is made non receptive to AIDS Virus by AUT and hyperthermia

Multiplication and Mutation of AIDS Virus (Fig. 11)

One of the problems encountered by the host immune system and vaccine producers is that the genome is quite variable. Certain regions of the virus are preserved while others show wide variation within the same individual, among groups of individuals and different geographic locations. This shows that the virus not only divides rapidly but somewhat carelessly, resulting in viral variations. This makes it difficult for the immune system to react effectively and is unable to recognize the specific viral antigen. That is why it may be difficult to make a vaccine against this virus. Scientists have recognized that gp-120 genetic material, a surface antigen, mutates very fast. These are the surface knobs that confront the immune system. According to Dr. Gerald Myers, director of the AIDS data base project at Los Alamos National lab in New Mexico, "the virus appears to be mutating millions of times faster than human DNA."

Presence of Cell-to-Cell Transmission of AIDS Virus

Until recently, efforts to develop an AIDS vaccine have been centered on the production of antibodies. These are capable of neutralizing the free virus before it infects the cell. Now it is becoming clear that the virus may be transmitted by direct cell-to-cell contact. According to Dr. Jay Levy of the University of California at San Francisco, "The most important mode of transmission from person to person is the virus infected cell." That is why it is difficult to transmit the AIDS virus from person to person. Infection occurs primarily by sexual contact, receiving contaminated blood, by using contaminated needles, and from an infected mother to a child in the womb or during birth.

The cell-to-cell contact mode of the AIDS virus spread also explains why a person develops AIDS even though they have neutralizing antibodies. These antibodies are supposed to control the free virus. Brain cells and fibroblasts infected with the AIDS virus (in vitro) do not have T4 receptors (T4 surface antigen) on them. This indicates the existence of additional unidentified receptors to which the AIDS virus becomes attached. During viral replication inside T4 cells, the viral glycoprotein may be incorporated into different areas of the cell membrane. This may disrupt the normal cell membrane and kill the infected cell. The viral envelop glycoprotein displayed on the infected cell may bind with the T4 receptor of a neighboring uninfected T4 cell. It then fuses with the cell wall complex, forming a syncytial cell. In this way one infected cell can kill up to 500 uninfected T4 cells. This results in massive T4 cell destruction, even though only a few of them are infected, according to Dr. William Hazeltine of Harvard's Dana-Farber Cancer Institute.

Dr. Robert C. Gallo of the National Cancer Institute does not totally agree with this concept. He contends that the infected cells act as reservoirs for the AIDS virus and transmit it to newly formal T4 helper/ inducer cells. AUT and hyperthermia eliminates cell to cell transmission of virus, syncytia formation, and destruction of non infected cells by infected cells.

The importance of finding cell-to-cell transmission is that any vaccine that has to be effective against the AIDS virus will have attack the virus infected cell reservoirs. The vaccine should elicit the immune cell's response. The immune system must recognize and kill infected cells in addition to eliciting neutralizing antibodies (Science, vol. 236, 24 April, 1981, p. 39-392).

According to Dr. Jay Levy, in those people who have the AIDS virus but have gone for a long time in good health, it would be difficult to remove the virus from the blood. When the suppressor T8 cells are removed, only then can you get the virus. Therefore, Dr. Levy thinks that the "suppressor T8 cells are keeping the virus in check." They may be doing this by producing antiviral agents such as interferon. Hyperthermia and AUT increases the number of T8 cells which keep the virus and virus infected cell under control without multiplication.

AIDS Virus Stores in the Body

Until now, it was believed that the HIV virus is found in AIDS patients, one in every 100,000 lymphocytes and monocytes. A new study published on December 14, 1989, in the New England Journal Medicine, by Dr.David D. Ho and his group at Ceder Sinai Medical Center, showed that at least one in 200 to 400 of these cells are infected with this virus. They also found that the virus produces new copies of itself which freely float outside the cells in blood plasma in people who are only HIV positive. These studies show that the virus does not lie dormant for years and the blood is very infective. This means that the contaminated syringe could carry anywhere from one half to 700 infective doses of this virus, depending on the stage of the disease.

New viruses in macrophages can hide inside a pocket called vacuoles located in the cell cytoplasm where the immune system cannot see it. Thus the virus thrives and survives protected from the immune system attack. A stimulus results in a high production of HIV. Freshly produced virus escapes from the infected cell and infects the healthy cells. Macrophages pass infection to other cells by touching and then fusing with them. Macrophages may be the main culprits in storing, protecting, and disseminating the HIV infection to other cells. AIDS dementia may be caused by substances released from the infected macrophages in the brain. HIV does not infect brain cells (in vivo). Experiments show that the gp 120, part from the surface of the AIDS virus can kill nerve cells. This provides a partial explanation for AIDs related dementia (Science News, vol. 134, 1988, p. 244).

Researchers have found that they are able to infect normal cells of the bone marrow (hematopoietic progenitor cells) with HIV in vitro. These cells are called mother blood cells because from them all other cells of the blood originate. This implies that the bone marrow may be a hidden reservoir of the virus in the body. Researchers have also shown that these cells can produce new virion without budding them off the cell membrane. They gather virus deep in the internal compartment (vacuoles and golgi complex) without being detected by the immune system. They do not display detectable CD4 surface receptor sites. The infected mother cells may account for some of the hematologic symptoms in many AIDS patients (myelodysplasia, leukopenia, various forms of cytopenia and anemia). Infected bone marrow cells continue to differentiate to produce infected monocytes and macrophages which also act as a reservoir. It looks as though the monocyte is the culprit and the lymphocyte is the innocent bystander.

The fibroblasts found all over the body can be infected even though they lack the CD_4 receptors. Thus the fibroblasts can also act as a reservoir for HIV in the body. HIV infected fibroblasts play a role in the connective tissue disorders seen in some HIV infected individuals (JAMA, 1989, vol. 261, p. 2999).

Tumor necrosis factor (TNF), a monokine secreted by the monocytes and macrophages, can trigger HIV viral replication. Interlukin-I alone has no such effect. How the TNF triggers viral replication is not known (JAMA, vol. 25, 1988, p. 3378). Any treatment designed to attack AIDS should take these facts into consideration; otherwise, the treatment is ineffective (Discover, Jan. 1989, p. 53).

Human Cells Susceptible to AIDS Virus Attack

This virus infects and hides in a wide array of cells in the human body besides T4 lymphocytes (JAMA, 1989, vol. 261, p. 2997-3006). AUT, hyperthermia with or without antimicrobial therapy reduces or eliminates AIDS Virus stores gradually. It may take long periods of AUT and up to six hyperthermia exposures or more to achieve total elimination of HIV stores in the body. Based on the studies, the following list of human cells are susceptible to HIV infections:

Hematopoietic Tissue
T-helper lymphocytes
B lymphocytes
Monocytes/macrophages
Promyelocyte
Dendritic cells
Stem cells in bone marrow

Nervous System
Astrocytes
Oligodendrocyte
Macrophages (microglia)
Capillary endothelial cells

Gastrointestinal Tract
Columnar and epithelial cells
Enterochromaffin cells
Colon carcinoma cells
Stromal macrophages and lymphocytes

Skin
Langerhans cells
Fibroblasts

Others
Osteosarcoma cells
Rhabdomyosarcoma cells
Kupffer's cells
Liver sinusoid epithelial cells
Fetal chorionic villi

Cofactors of HIV Infection in the Development of AIDS

It has been shown that HIV does not reproduce in resting lymphocyte in the laboratory. Activated lymphocytes from normal donors has to be added in order to cultivate the virus in vitro. This suggest that certain factors are needed to activate the virus inside our body. These factors are called co-factors. Use of inhalation nitrites, herpes simplex virus, cytomegalo virus, hepatitis B virus, Epstein barr virus, human T cell lymphotrophic virus, amebiasis, giardiasis, syphilis and sexually transmitted diseases, environmental toxins including alcohol, opiates, marijuana, stress, physical trauma, malnutrition, can all play a role in disease progression and act as co-factors.

Recently, Shyh-Ching Lo, M.D., and associates of the Armed Forces Institute of Pathology have reported a virus-like infectious agent (VLIA) from seven AIDS donor cells. They inoculated four silver-head leaf monkeys with VLIA. All of them died within nine months with severe weight loss and low-grade fever. Examination of tissue from these monkeys showed VLIA in the brain, liver, and spleen cells. If these findings are proved, this VLIA becomes a co-factor to the HIV. VLIA operates in collusion with HIV to speed progression from HIV infection to clinical disease. This supports the group of investigators who claim that HIV alone does not cause AIDS. Studies are in progress to prove these findings one way or the other (JAMA, 1989, vol. 261, no. 23, p. 3361-3362, Am J. Trop Med. Hyg., 1989, vol. 40, pp. 213-226, 399-409). Recently at the fifth international conference in Montreal, Canada, Dr. Robert C. Gallo suggested HHV-6 virus, which infects a large population, might act as a catalyst that causes HIV to reproduce in human cells (AMA News, July 28, 1989). Mycoplasma organism, syphilis and many other unknown factors have also been blamed as cofactors in the development of AIDS.

AIDS: A World Wide Health Problem

All European and Asian countries have reported AIDS. According to WHO estimates 8 million people are infected with AIDS virus and more than 20 millions will be infected all over the world by the end of this decade. One in 40 adult men and women are infected with HIV in sub-Saharan Africa. In latin America, there are 500,000 HIV positive with 22,000 AIDS cases. In India and Thailand, as many as half a million people are infected. Most of the African countries spend less than $7.00 per person per year on health care. HIV positive test ranges from 2 to 50% in Central Africa. In Rawanda it is 10% and Zaire, 15%. Sexual promiscuity, multiple sexual partners among homosexuals, and frequent contact with prostitutes in heterosexuals play major roles in spread of the disease. For example, 54% of Kenyan and 80% of Rawanda prostitutes were HIV positive. In another study, 18% of blood donors in Lusaka (Zambia), 7% of the population of Kinshasha City (Zaire), a city of 4 million, and 67% of prostitutes of Nairobi (Kenya) are tested positive (AIDS Guide for Survival, 1988, p. 17). Studies in Rawanda indicate that 75% of the male patients with AIDS reported frequent and regular sexual contact with different partners, including prostitutes.

The male-to-female ratio of AIDS in the United States is 15:1. In Africa, it is 1:1 in Zaire, Rawanda, Kinshasha, and Kigali. This data supports the spread of AIDS from male to female and vice versa. According to World Health Organization (WHO), millions of

Africans will die from AIDS and its related disease by the year 2000. Ignorance about the disease and its mode of spread is said to be responsible for such a massive spread of the disease in Africa.

Who Gets AIDS?

Analysis of the origin and spread of HIV shows that AIDS is not a disease of homosexuals, drug addicts or any particular risk group. It is not God-sent either to punish gays. The virus is spread by intimate contact. The type and form of contact is less important compared to the contact itself. In Africa, the AIDS pool is made up primarily of heterosexuals. Whereas in America, homosexuals and drug abusers comprise most patients in the pool. It is transmitted from mother to child during pregnancy. Many children born to intravenous drug abusers are positive for HIV tests. This virus has been isolated from the organs of a 20-week fetus after an abortion in a HIV positive IV drug user. In Australia mothers were infected by artificial insemination from an infected donor. The infants born to these mothers were free of the disease. Breast milk does contain the AIDS virus in HIV positive women. Seven HIV negative mothers who breast fed HIV positive babies developed AIDS in Elista, Russia. Breast feeding should be avoided if mother or child is HIV positive.

Everyone is at risk in contracting AIDS. Getting AIDS has nothing to do with whether you are homo-, hetero-, or bisexual, or whether you are white, black, brown, or yellow, or whether you are young or old, rich or poor. As Dr. June Osborne, Dean of the School of Public Health at the University of Michigan contends, "It is not who you are but what you do" (U.S. News & World Report, Jan. 12, 1987). The cost of careless sex can be your life.
Gay and bisexual men account for 65% of AIDS cases in the United States, and 8% are IV drug abusers.

There are 13 million units of blood transfused every year in U.S. As of 1986, 316 cases of AIDS have been linked to contaminated blood and its products. There are reports of many infants developing AIDS due to use of contaminated blood needles in Romania. Of the approximate 17,000 hemophiliacs in the United States, the incidence is 3.6 per 1000 hemophiliac A patients and 0.6

per 1000 hemophiliac B patients. There are 360 known cases of AIDS victims who are under the age of 13, 60% of which have died.

Transmission from women to women (lesbian) is rare. It is possible only if they engage in oral/genital, and oral/anal sex. Hepatitis and other sexually transmitted diseases are spread through these sexual modes. French kissing should be avoided with partners whose health is in question and if one does not know a partners sexual history. There are no cases of HIV spread through saliva but it can occur. However, some diseases are spread through saliva and contact with saliva should be avoided.

Evidence for AIDS spread by mosquitos, handshakes, toilet seats, tears, saliva, sneezing, sweat, coughing, hugging, contact with eating utensils, swimming pools, gymnasiums, telephones, typewriters, computers, water fountains, being close to other people as in crowded places (buses, office, classroom, games, etc.), is lacking. Needle sticks do transmit the AIDS virus. Transmission of AIDS by patient bites does exists. Such risky behavior should be discouraged.

Seven cases of AIDS were reported from Elista Russia. The virus was transmitted from HIV positive babies to their mothers during breast feeding. Seventy-three children developed AIDS in Elista and Volgogard of Russia by the careless use of contaminated needles (A.M.A.News, June 16, 1989, p. 11). This shows the importance of using sterile techniques while handling body fluids and blood from AIDS patients.

Health Care Workers and AIDS

Thirty persons, including physicians, who provided health care to AIDS patients or came in contact with the contaminated material have developed HIV positive test. Four of those cases followed needle stick exposure to the blood from patients infected with HIV. Two other cases did not have needle sticks but had extensive contact with infected patients' blood and fluids. There are 50 to 100 HIV infectious particles per ml of plasma or semen compared to 100 million to 1 billion infectious particles per ml of hepatitis B virus.

That is why the spread of HIV by needle stick injury is low compared to hepatitis.

The CDC has also learned of additional health care worker following non-needle sticks. A female health care worker had blood spattered on her chapped hands during an arterial stick on an AIDS patient with a cardiac arrest. She did not wash for twenty minutes, and she tested HIV positive 16 weeks after exposure. The second health care worker is a phlebotomist who had blood spattered on her face and mouth. She had facial acne and had no needle stick or open wound. She became positive nine months later. The other worker is a female who had blood splattered on her hand and forearm while handling a blood component separation device. She had dermatitis of the ear and may have scratched this area with contaminated hands. She became HIV positive in three months (JAMA, June 12, 1987, vol. 257, 2, p. 3032). None of these people were wearing gloves and did not follow CDC recommended guidelines.

Recently (July 1990) CDC reported a case of possible transfer of AIDS virus from a HIV positive dentist working on molar teeth of a healthy female. This case raises the possibility of AIDS spread by droplets. Health care proveders should guard against getting infection from patients during washing, using mechnical equipments, secretions, blood etc. by contact and droplets.

The HIV can spread by coming in contact with open wounds or mucous membranes or needle sticks. If the health care worker has an open wound, he/she should avoid working with infected blood and patients. If there is no choice, strict preventive precautions should be followed. Each time a health care worker suffers a needle stick injury, he has a 1 in 2000 chance of contacting AIDS if he is treating an AIDS patient. In areas where there are few HIV positive patients, the chances of contacting AIDS from needle sticks are 1 in 200,000 (AMA News, January 13, 1989, p. 20).

All health care workers should wear gloves and protective goggles. Do not cap the needle while handling AIDS patients and drawing their blood. A recent study from the Ceder Sinai from Los Angeles (NEJM, December 14, 1989) showed that a contaminated syringe could carry one half to 700 infective doses of the virus, depending on the stage of infection. Those who are exposed should undergo AUT and dry sauna treatment as described in hyperthermia chapters to eliminate HIV before it establishes a foot hold.

AIDS in the Newborn

Mothers can transmit the virus to their first child 25% to 50% of the time and 65% of the time if she gives birth to a first infected child. Diagnosis of HIV infection in children born to the infected mother is hampered by the presence of maternal antibody to HIV during the first fifteen months of life. Diagnosis of HIV infection in child may be the first indication that the mother and the other members of the family are infected. Disease is expressed within 3-24 months. Child may remain asymptomatic up to age of seven. Symptoms such as enlarged liver, spleen and lymph nodes, failure to thrive, chronic diarrhea, oral thrush, recurrent viral and bacterial infections, cardiomyopathy, renal diseases and encephalopathy (weakness of limbs, loss of developmental milestones) all indicate AIDS.

Dr. Kubler-Ross, author of *Death and Dying*, aside from her own out-of-body experiences, falsely claimed that she has "Cured AIDS in 2 children by love alone" (Atlanta meeting on February 12, 1990). She led the audience to believe that these two children had AIDS. However, they were only positive due to antibodies transferred from their mother during pregnancy. They became negative after a lapse of time since there was no real HIV infection.

Different Sexual Practices and Risk of AIDS

Safe sexual practices

1. Massage, hugging, cuddling
2. Mutual masturbation
3. Social kissing (dry)
4. Body-to-body rubbing (frottage)
5. Voyeurism, exhibitionism, fantasy

Possibly safe, still dangerous
1. Tongue kissing
2. Vaginal intercourse with condom
3. Anal intercourse with condom
4. Cunnilingus
5. Fellatio without condom, stopping before climax (can be unsafe also)

Unsafe sex all the time
1. Vaginal intercourse without condom with unknown partners
2. Anal intercourse without condom
3. Blood contact (including menstrual blood)
4. Fellatio without condom; semen or urine in mouth
5. Anilingus ("rimming")
6. Hand in rectum ("fisting")
7. Sharing sex toys and needles that had contact with body fluids

Sex During Menstruation and Chances of AIDS infection

Sex during menstruation increases the risk of female to male transmission. Because:
1. It will bring men in direct contact with blood potentially infected with AIDS virus.
2. In most women during active menstruation, that the cells capable of hosting HIV are secreted from the cervix (JAMA 264: 333, 1990).

Avoid having sex during monthly periods with high risk group. Use of nonoxynol-9 sponge is not good enough. It is possible that the repeated use of this spermicide can irritate cervical mucosa resulting in lymphocyte infiltration. Some of these lymphocytes can be loaded with AIDS virus which can infect male partners. Use of double condoms is the safest approach, if you engage in sex during menstruation.

Diseases Transmitted by Artificial Insemination

There are about 60,000 women who have been artificially inseminated became pregnant and had a baby. There are untold numbers of women who were inseminated but did not get pregnant or carry the pregnancy to completion. These women should be aware that many kinds of disease-causing organisms such as Neisseria gonorrhea, trichomonas vaginalis, urea plasma urealyticum, mycoplasma hominis, AIDS virus, chlamydia trachomatic and streptococcal species, and hepatitis B virus have been transmitted from donor semen to inseminated women. All donors for these cases were asymptomatic at the time of semen donation (JAMA, Feb. 27, 1987, vol. 257, p. 1093-94). Hyperthermia and AUT can eliminate sexually transmitted diseases.

Myths: Can Some People Not Get AIDS at All?

Even today we do not know why some people, in spite of repeated exposure, do not get the HIV infection. There are many who do not show symptoms of illness for a long time after infection. Many scientist believe that traumatic sexual intercourse, such as "anal sex," causes damage to mucous membranes and blood vessels. This allows the virus to enter the blood stream directly and easily. On the other hand, there is a report of getting AIDS by artificial insemination. Trauma to the genital area is not the only factor in the transmission of AIDS. It is also possible that genetic make up plays a role. The gene-controlled surface protein located in the T4 lymphocytes makes it easier or harder to spread the disease. That is why AIDS is high in blacks and Hispanics (24% of AIDS cases which make up 12% of the U.S. population) compared to the white population. It is spreading like wild fire in Africa. According to Dr. Stephen Daiger of Medical Genetic Department of the University of Texas Health Science Center at Houston, the GC-1 fast gene which increases the susceptibility is found more frequently in African blacks than caucasians. Hepatitis C virus is found in higher percentage of blacks and spanish population with AIDS. What role it play in production AIDS, we do not know.

FIGURE 11: SHOWS STRUCTURE, GENETIC MAKEUP AND LIFE CYCLE OF AIDS VIRUS INSIDE HOST CELL AND ITS MECHANISM OF REPRODUCTION.

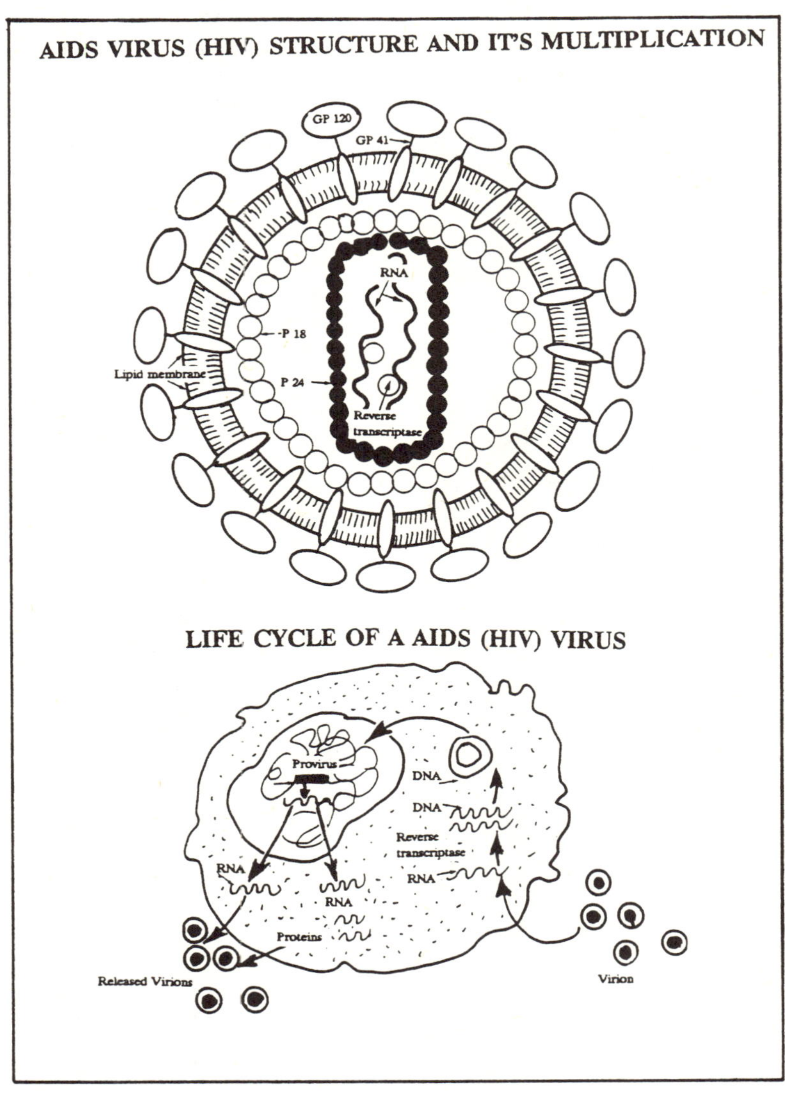

FIGURE 12: SHOWS THE DESTRUCTION OF T4 CELLS BY AIDS VIRUS.

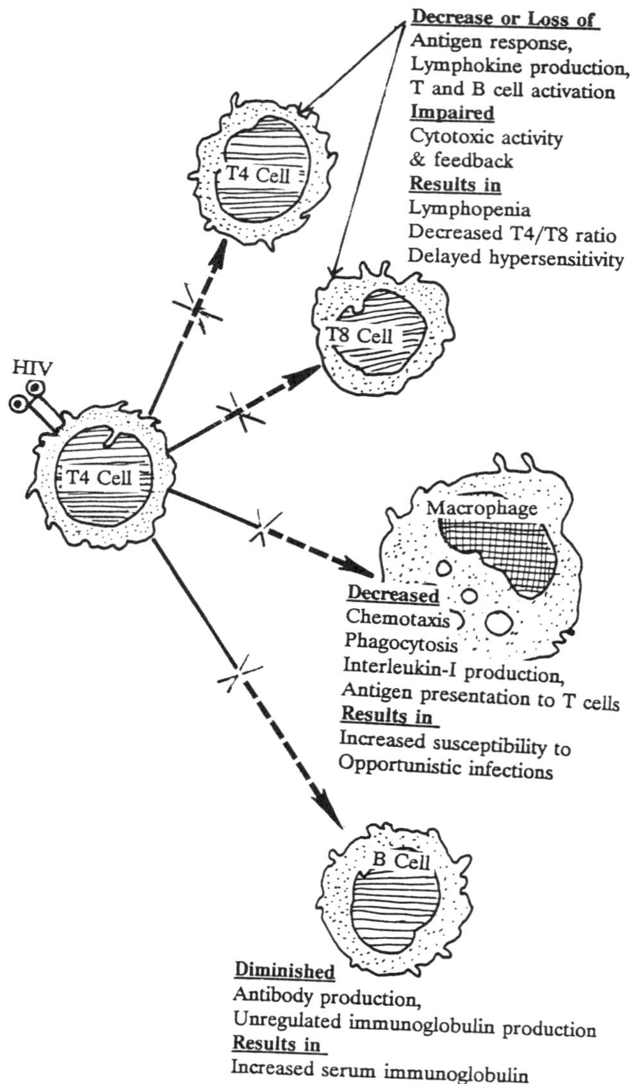

FIGURE 13: SHOWING THE INFECTION OF T4 CELLS BY AIDS VIRUS (HIV) AND THEIR DESTRUCTION

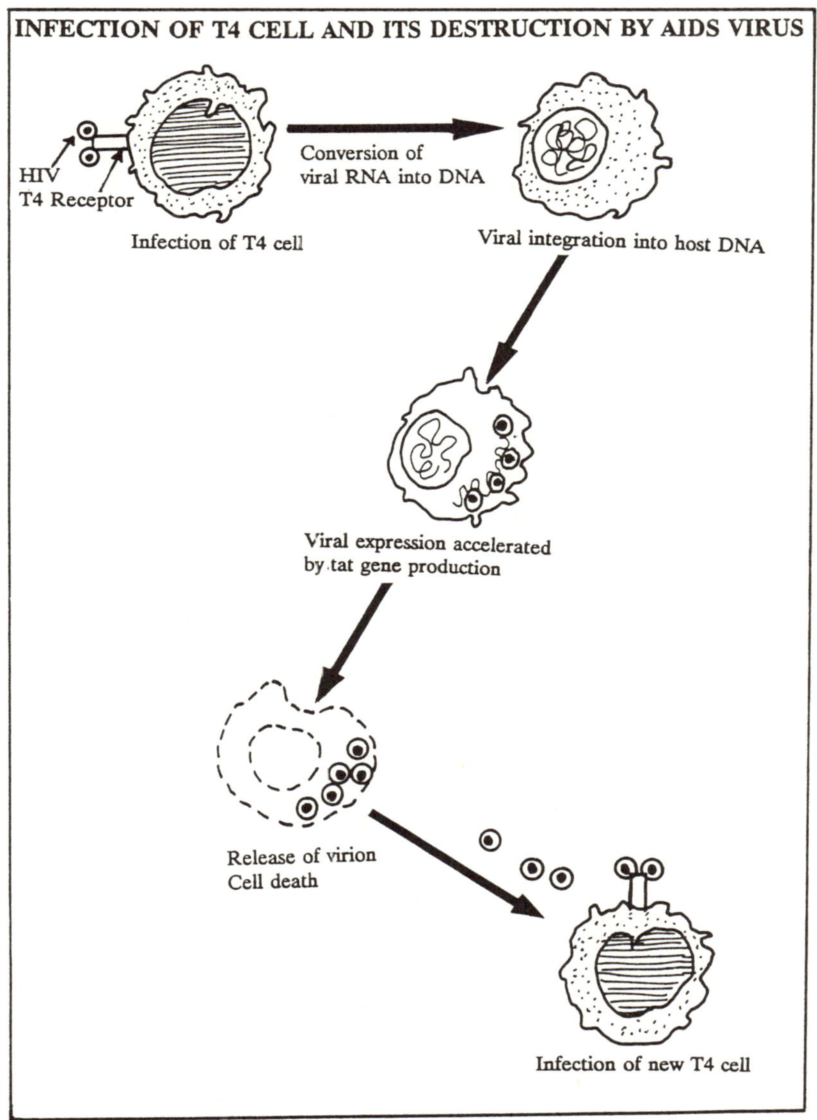

CHAPTER 16

AIDS - CLINICAL ASPECTS

Signs and Symptoms

Today my body is in eclipse,
when is the release,
O'Lord of the meeting rivers?
Basaveswara
12th Century Shiva Saint from India

Definition

In the United States, the CDC defines a case of "acquired immunodeficiency syndrome" (AIDS) as an illness characterized by:

1. One or more opportunistic diseases diagnosed by methods considered reliable (histology, cytology, endoscopic examination, or culture). The disease is moderately indicative of cellular immunodeficiency (Table I).

2. Absence of all known underlying causes of cellular immunodeficiency other than HTLV-III (HIV) infection and absence of all other causes of reduced resistance reported to be associated with at least one of those opportunistic diseases (Table II).

Despite having the above criteria, patients are excluded from an AIDS diagnosis if the are negative for antibody to HIV, do not have a positive culture for HIV, and have a normal or high number of T4-helper lymphocytes. In the absence of test results, patients satisfying all other criteria in this definition are included as AIDS cases.

TABLE I - Diseases at Least Moderately Indicative of Cellular Immunodeficiency

(Source: CDC Case Definition of AIDS)

1. Kaposi's sarcoma.
2. Pneumocystic carinii pneumonia (PCP).
3. Toxoplasmosis infection of internal organs other than liver, spleen, or lymph nodes.
4. Cryptosporidiosis intestinal, causing diarrhea over a month.
5. Candidiasis, causing esophagitis.
6. Cryptosporidiosis, causing central nervous system or other infections disseminated beyond the lungs and lymph nodes.
7. Mycobacterium avium or intracellular (Mycobacterium avium complex) causing infection disseminated beyond the lungs and lymph nodes.
8. Primary lymphoma of the brain.
9. Progressive multifocal leukoencephalopathy (Papova virus infection of the brain).
10. Chrnic mucocutaneous herpes simplex infection ulcers persisting more than one month.

TABLE II - Known Causes of Reduced Resistance

(Source: CDC Case Definition of AIDS)

1. Systemic corticosteroid therapy.
2. Other immunosuppressive or cytotoxic therapy.
3. Cancer of lymphoreticular or histiocytic tissue, such as lymphoma (except for lymphoma localized to the brain), Hodgkin's disease, lymphocytic leukemia, or multiple myeloma.
4. Age 60 years or older at diagnosis.
5. Age under 28 days (neonatal at diagnosis).
6. Age under 6 months at diagnosis.
7. Immunodeficiency atypical of AIDS, such as one involving hypogamma-globulinemia or angioimmunoblastic

lymphadenopathy; or an immuno-deficiency of which the cause appears to be a genetic or developmental defect rather than HIV infection.

8. Exogenous malnutrition (due to starvation, not due to malnutrition but due to malabsorption or illness).

CDC Classification of AIDS Virus Infection

There is a full range of conditions and syndromes associated with AIDS. In May, 1986, the CDC issued a comprehensive classification of systems for categorizing patients infected with HIV. (CDC's M. M. R 35, 334, 1986). The Walter Reed Army Institute of Research also reported a classification based on clinical and laboratory parameters. The following summarizes the classification described by the CDC.

Group I: Acute Infection

Mononucleosis-like syndrome associated with sero-conversion.

Group II: Asymptomatic Infection

Positive HIV antibody or viral culture. May be subclassified on basis of laboratory evaluation (CBC, platelet count, T-cell subset studies).

Group III: Persistent Generalized Lymphadenopathy

Palpable lymph node enlargement (> 1cm) at two or more extra inguinal (groin) sites for more than three months without a concurrent illness or infection to explain the findings. May be subclassified on the basis of laboratory evaluation (see above).

Group IV - Other HIV Disease

Subgroup A: Constitutional Disease

One or more of the following: fever or diarrhea persisting more than one month or involuntary weight loss greater than 10% of baseline; and absence of a concurrent illness or infection to explain the findings.

Subgroup B: Neurologic Disease
One or more of the following: dementia, myelopathy, or peripheral neuropathy; and absence of a concurrent illness or condition.

Subgroup C: Secondary Infectious Diseases
Infectious disease associated with HIV infection and/or least moderately indicative of a defect in cell-mediated immunity.

Category C-1
Symptomatic or invasive disease due to one of 12 specified diseases listed in the surveillance definition of AIDS: Pneumocystis carinii pneumonia, chronic cryptosporidiosis, toxoplasmosis, extra intestinal strongyloidiasis, isosporiasis, candidiasis (esophageal, bronchial, or pulmonary), cryptococcoses, histoplasmosis, mycobacterial infection (Mycobacterium avium complex or M. kansasii), cytomegalovirus infection, chronic mucocutaneous or disseminated herpes simplex virus infection, and progressive multifocal leukoencephalopathy.

Category C-2
Symptomatic or invasive disease due to one of six other specified diseases: oral hairy leukoplakia, multidermatomal herpes zoster, recurrent Salmonella bacteremia, nocardiosis, tuberculosis, and oral candidiasis (thrush).

Subgroup D: Secondary Cancers
Diagnosis of one or more cancers known to be associated with HIV infection as listed in the surveillance definition of AIDS and at least moderately indicative of a defect in cell-mediated immunity: Kaposi sarcoma, non-Hodgkin's lymphoma (small, noncleaved lymphoma or immunoblastic sarcoma), or primary lymphoma of the brain.

Subgroup E: Other Conditions in HIV Infection
Clinical findings or disease, not classifiable above, that may be attributable to HIV infection and are indicative of a defect in cell mediated immunity; symptoms attributable to either HIV infection or a coexisting disease not classified elsewhere; or clinical illnesses that may be complicated or altered by HIV infection. These include chronic lymphoid interstitial pneumonitis and constitutional symptoms, secondary infectious diseases, and neoplasms not listed above of AIDS which takes into account newly recognized symptoms such as "AIDS related dementia" and weight loss known as "wasting syndrome. "

Walter Reed's Classification of AIDS

The Walter Reed (WR) Classification System charts the course of patients from exposure to HIV (WR0) and the onset of infection (WR1) through stages of progressive immune dysfunction. Based on laboratory evidence of HIV infection, Stage 2 is characterized by swollen lymph nodes and Stage 3 is reached when the T4-cell count drops below 400 cells per cubic millimeter of blood and stays down (normal count is > 800). A patient moves into Stage 4 after sub-clinical (asymptomatic) defects are found in delayed hypersensitivity. The ability to react to skin tests that are a barometer of immune functioning ("P" indicates a partial defect). Stage 5 the patient completely ("C") fails to respond to the skin test or when thrush (a fungal disease of the mouth) develops (Lymphadenopathy and abnormalities of T4 cell and skin test must persist for at least three months to serve as criteria). Patients enter Stage 6 and are said to have AIDS when opportunistic infections develop because the immune system has broken down (N. Engl. J. Med, 314, 132, 1985).

TABLE OF WALTER REED CLASSIFICATION SYSTEM OF AIDS

Stage	HIV antibody or virus isolation	Chronic lymphadenopathy	T- helper cells / cubic mm	Delayed hypersensitivity	Thrush	Opportunistic infections
WR-0	-	-	>400	N	-	-
WR-1	+	-	>400	N	-	-
WR-2	+	+	<400	N	-	-
WR-3	+	±	<400	N	-	-
WR-4	+	±	<400	P	-	-
WR-5	+	±	<400	C	+	-
WR-6	+	±	<400	P/C	±	+

N=Normal, P=Partial cutaneous anergy, C=complete cutaneous anergy

Clinical Signs and Symptoms of HIV Infection

Symptoms mimicking infectious mononucleosis

Fever
Pharyngitis (sore throat)
Lymphadenopathy (lymph gland swelling)
Arthralgia, myalgia (pains all over)
Headache, pain behind the eye balls
Lethargy, malaise (Weakness)
Loss of weight and appetite
Nausea, vomiting
Diarrhea

Nervous system disorders

Meningitis
Encephalitis
Peripheral neuropathy
Radiculopathy
Gullain-Barre syndrome
Cognitive or affective impairment

Skin conditions

Erythematous maculopapular rash
Roseola like rash
Diffuse urticaria
Skin peeling (Desquamation)
Alopecia (loss of hairs in spots)
Palate or gum ulceration

Review of Systems for Potential Signs and Symptoms of HIV Infection

1. **General examination and history taking:** Weight loss, anorexia, fever, sweats.
2. **Skn:** pruritus, rashes or pigmented lesions, drying and peeping of skin.
3. **Lymphatic:** Lymph node enlargement, change in size or increase in size of the lymph nodes.

4. **Head, eyes, ears, nose, and throat:** Headaches, nasal discharge, sinus congestion, sore throat, whitish or painful lesions of the oral mucosa, change in vision.
5. **Cardiopulmonary:** Cough or shortness of breath, increased heart rate, finger tip ashy color.
6. **Gastrointestinal:** Abdominal pain, loss of appetite, change in bowel habits, diarrhea.
7. **Musculoskeletal:** Muscle and joint pain.
8. **Nerologic:** Change in personality, cognitive difficulties, symptoms of depression, change of personality, bowel or bladder dysfunction, peripheral nerve weakness or paresthesia.

Earliest Stages of HIV Infection

Some people remain healthy after infection with the AIDS virus and do not show any clear-cut symptoms. These are the people who think they are free from the disease despite their high risk behavior and can spread the virus to other people. Respect other human beings. If you are involved in risky behavior, wait six months before you have sex with another, innocent healthy partner. Get tested every six weeks for six months before you claim yourself safe and free of AIDS virus. The median incubation period for developing AIDS is 30 months in adults and 16 months in children.

At the earliest stages, HIV infection resembles infectious mononucleosis, colds and flu. It is characterized by fever, sweats, muscle pain, joint pains, sore throat, lethargy, weakness, anorexia, nausea, vomiting, headache, and occasionally diarrhea. Initially, the HIV test is negative, and becomes positive usually within six months. Now there are tests being developed which can detect AIDS within 48 hour after exposure. If you belong to high-risk group and develop the above symptoms, do get tested for HIV every six weeks. Avoid sex with other partners for at least six months until the repeated tests are negative. The HIV infection may be associated with neurologic symptoms (encephalopathy) that subside spontaneously. This infection may be associated with persistent lymph node swelling.

Summary of AIDS Symptoms

1. Unexplained fever, night sweats, and chills lasting many weeks.
2. Persistent and unexplained fatigue.
3. Unexplained weight loss (more than 10 lbs).
4. Persistent dry cough.
5. Severe weakness.
6. Diarrhea.
7. White hairy spots of the mouth and tongue lasting several weeks.
8. Lymph node swelling all over the body.

AIDS-Related Complex (ARC)

ARC patients are a group of patients who are positive for HIV antibody and have generalized lymph node swelling, persistent low grade fever, unexplained weight loss, and diarrhea. They may also have tuberculosis, oral thrush, hairy leukoplakia on tongue (white patch on tongue), herpes zoster, neuropathy (central and peripheral), dementia due to encephalitis, and cerebral lymphoma. This may be associated with many opportunistic infections. The CDC classification of group III and IV and subgroups A and B falls into the definition of ARC.

What to Look for if You Suspect HIV Infection

1. Unique to HIV infection

Hairy leukoplakia on the tongue
Disseminated Kaposi's sarcoma

2. Suggestive of HIV (other immunodeficiency states excluded)

Cytomegalovirus retinitis(eye infection)
Oral (mouth) candidiasis

3. Commonly found but not specific to HIV infection

a. Skin conditions: xerosis, tinea, folliculitis, psoriasis, onycholysis
b. Eyes: cotton wool spots
c. Mouth cavity: Aphthous and herpetic esions

d. Lymphatic: Lymph node enlargement, other than the groin glands
e. Abdomen: Liver and Spleen enlargement
f. Neurologic: Decreased global cognition, psychomotor slowing, ataxia, changes in reflexes (hypo- or hyper), hypesthesia
g. Psychiatric: Depression, mania, psychosis

Autoantibodies Produced in AIDS and the Diseases They Produce: Immune Defense Response of the Host to AIDS Virus Infection

This viral infection produces immune responses both beneficial and detrimental to the host. The first reaction of the host is lymphocyte B proliferation; this is, due to stimulation by HIV envelope glycoprotein. It results in an increase in gamma globulin. This increase in immunoglobulin production leads to autoimmune syndromes, that is antibodies produced against normal cellular proteins in the body. This happens because many of the AIDS viral parts resemble cellular proteins (such as interferon, HLA antigen, Interlukin-II, alpha thymosin, neuroleukin, peptide T). Many auto-antibodies act against the following host cells, producing appropriate diseases. (JAMA 1989, vol. 261, p. 3002).

HIV infection also leads to production of neutralizing antibodies which act against the HIV and its transfer to other cells. These antibodies act only on selected HIV strains. This shows there are several types of HIV. To be effective, a vaccine must contain different serological groups of HIV and antibodies. Antibodies also help kill infected cells by coating and marking them for destruction by the hosts' effector cells. In AIDS patients, the virus can induce the production of antibodies that enhance the viral infection. This probably helps speed the spread of HIV infection and its effects leading to AIDS.

The human body produce T8 lymphocytes. These T8 cells attack and kill the HIV infected cells. This killing effect is said to be directed against HIV gag, pol, and env protein expressed on the surface of infected cells. The HIV infected individuals also produce T8 cells that are endowed with the capacity to suppress virus production in infected cells. This is said to be due to production of lymphokine by T8 cells.

Cells Affected in AIDS and Diseases Produced

1. **Platelets:** Thrombocytopenic purpura (bleeding)
2. **Red blood cells:** Anemia (look pale, weak)
3. **Neutrophilc:** Neutropenia (easy infection)
4. **Peripheral nerves:** Neuropathy (numbness and tingling)
5. **Lymphocyte:** Immune deficiency (Infections)
6. **Lupus anticoagulant:** Thrombosis (blood clot formation)
7, **Phospholipids:** Neurologic disease (see the list)
8. **Nucleus (ANA):** Autoimmunity (ANA = Antinuclear antibody)

All these cells affected by the AIDS Virus are replaced by new cells by AUT and hyperthermia

Immunological abnormalities seen in AIDS

1. **Abnormalities in T cells**
   CD4 cell depletion
   Decrease proliferation of soluble antigens
   Decreased helper response for PWM induced immunoglobulin synthesis
   Impaired or delayed-type hypersensitivity
   Decreased alpha interferon production in response to antigens
   Reduced proliferation to T-cell mitogens, alloantigens and to anti-CD4
   Decreased AMLR response
   Lower cell-mediated cytotoxicity to virally infected cells
   Decreased IL-2 production
   Decreased in Lymphocytes

2. **Abnormalities in B cells**
   Polyclonal activation with hyper gammaglobulinemia (IgG, IgA, and lgd), increased spontaneous plaque forming cells and proliferation
   Decreased humoral response to immunization
   Circulating autoantibodies

3. Abnormalities in Macrophages and monocytes
Decreased chemotaxis

4. Abnormalities in natural killer cells
Decreased cytotoxicity

5. Other immune responses
Increased acid-labile alpha-interferon production
Increased soluble immune complexes
Decreased alpha-1 thymosin

Most of the immune system abnormalities are corrected by AUT and hyperthermia.

Other Diseases That Have to be Differentiated from HIV Infection

1. Epstein-Barr virus mononucleosis
2. Cytomegalovirus mononucleosis, toxoplasmosis
3. Rubella
4. Viral hepatitis
5. Syphilis
6. Widespread gonococcal infection
7. Herpes simplex virus
8. Other viral infections
9. Drug reactions

Indicators of AIDS Progression: Symptoms and Signs

1. Continued Fevers
2. Weght loss > 10 per cent of normal body weight
3. Persistent diarrhea
4. Mental disorders - Cognitive changes-Encephalopathy
5. History of Herpes zoster, candidiasis, hairy leukoplakia
6. Anemia
7. Elevated erythrocyte sedimentation rate
8. Decreased T4- lymphocytes
9. Persistent generalized lymph node enlargement (without other findings, has better outlook)

After autoimmune urine therapy and hyperthermia, these symptoms of progression are reversed.

Kaposi's Sarcoma and Other Tumors

Other pathology seen in AIDS is the development of cancers such as Kaposi's sarcoma, cancer of the mouth, skin, rectum and B cell lymphoma arising from B lymphocytes. It has been experimentally shown that the that gene from HIV can produce tumors in mice, suggesting that the AIDS virus is a cancer causing virus (Science News, vol. 143, 1978, p. 244; Nature Oct. 13, 1988). It has also been thought that the depression of the immune system enables secondary tumor causing agents to infect and replicate freely, thereby causing cancer.

I believe that Kaposi tumor is not a true sarcoma. It is resulting from immune system reaction and can be eliminated by hyperthermia and AUT. About 25% of the AIDS patients develop Kaposi's sarcoma. It is characterized by slow growing dark brown or purple blue nodules or plaques found all over the body, but predominantly on the legs. The lungs, digestive system, and lymphatic system can also show these lesions. These lesions look like a vascular neoplasm containing vascular elements embedded in spindle cells. The median survival for those AIDS patients presenting with Kaposi's sarcoma is 125 weeks. Where as with PCP pneumonia it is only 48 weeks. With advancement in treatment, longevity of these patients is increasing. Kaposi's sarcoma is treated with radiation (for bulky Kaposis), alpha interferon, chemotherapeutic agents, (AZT, doxorubicin, vinblastine, bleomycin, dactinomycin, vincristine, decambizine), etc. Hyperthermia by radiant heat, dry sauna, hot water tubs, hot jacuzzi, AUT can eliminate Kaposi sarcoma or decrease their chances of development.

Brain and Spinal Cord Infection

It is thought that the infected monocytes and macrophages, a kind of white blood cells, carry the virus to the brain and spinal cord. The virus and host cell products have a direct disease-causing effect on the brain and spinal cord and is not dependent on immune deficiency. There is abnormal proliferation of cells surrounding nerve cells (glial cells). This results in loss of white matter. The viral invasion of the nervous system gives rise to a wide range of symptoms, including dementia. It may mimic many brain and spinal cord diseases including multiple sclerosis. There is evidence showing that GP-120 of the AIDS virus can kill nerve cells. The whole virus is not needed to cause damage to the brain. See the table for AIDS complications of the nervous system. AUT and hyperthermia relieves the brain and spinal cord afflictions of AIDS Virus.

The latest report indicates that the AIDS dementia may be linked to a metabolite of Tryptophan (JAMA 264:305-306. 1990). Quinolinic acid is a neurotoxic convulsant metabolite of tryptophan activated by interferon gamma. It raises as much as 1000 folds in AIDS patients with dementia. It is also elevated after common cold virus to lenti virus infections. It is likely most of the viral infections including rabies, it is increased contributing to mental symptoms. "Can't think properly" during cold can be attributed to this metabolite associated mental changes. It binds to nerve receptors (N-methyl-D-aspartate receptors) which are involved in normal neurotransmission, neural regulation, memory, and synaptic plasticity. It can also induce seizures and nerve cell death. The levels of these metabolites go up with dementia and opportunistic infections of the central nervous system such as toxoplasmosis, progressive multifocal leukoencephalopathy, lymphomas, etc. The enzyme (indoleamine-2, -3-dioxygenase, IDL) which converts tryptophan to quinolinic acid increases in the lungs and brain. So the metabolism shifts from the liver to brain. Hyperthermia breaks the blood brain barrier. With AUT, it flushes out all the quinolinic acid and neutralizes the IDL enzyme which converts tryptophan into this toxic substance. Hyperthermia and AUT will reduce or eliminate AIDS or other infection associated dementia including AIDS and rabies.

Various Systemic Manifestations of AIDS

The list is growing every day and looks endless.

1. **Skin conditions**

   Herpes Zoster, and simplex

Erythematous rash
Generalized pruritus
Seborrheic dermatitis
Psoriasis
Trichophyton rubrum
Molluscum contagiosum
Miliaria
Candidiasis
Tenia pedis and facie

2. **Oral (mouth) manifestations**
Oral candidiasis
Hairy Leukoplakia
Kaposi's sarcoma
Herpes simplex infection
Papillomas
Gingivitis

3. **Gastrointestinal manifestations**
Esophagitis due to Candida, CMV, herpes infection, hepatitis due to cytomegalo virus, mycobacterium avium and intracellulare (MAI), CMV, and other infections
Gastroenteritis due to MAI, crytosporidium isospora, salmonella, shigella, campylobacter, adenovirus infections, etc.
Chronic malabsorption syndrome associates with diarrhea, and steatorrhea

4. **Eye manifestations**
Cytomegalo virus (CMV)
Chorioretinitis
Toxoplasmosis retinitis
Fungal and bacterial endophthalmitis
Kaposi's sarcoma of the eyelids

5. **Neurologic manifestations**
Peripheral neuropathy
Diffuse encephalitis

Paraplegia, brain hemorrhage, stroke
Behavioral mental changes
Dementia
Central nervous system (CNS) infection by Toxoplasmosis, cryptococcoses, fungal and bacterial brain abscess
Lymphoma
Meningitis (Bacterial, tubercular, fungal, viral)

6. **Cardiac complications**
Myocarditis due to cryptococcoses, toxoplasmosis, CMV infection
Pericardial kaposi, sarcoma
Pericarditis

7. **Pulmonary complications**
Pneumocystic carinii pneumonia (PCP)
Cytomegalovirus (CMV) infection
Pulmonary tuberculosis
Legionella
Cryptococcus
Kaposi's sarcoma
Other forms of pneumonia

8. **Renal complications**
Nephrotic type proteinuria
Azotemia
Renal failure due to segmental glomerulosclerosis

9. **Blood related (Hematologic) changes**
Lymphocytosis
Lowered T4 lymphocytes
Increase in T8 cells
Anemia
Myelofibrosis of bone marrow
Wide-spread disruption of blood forming elements
Bleeding due to low platelets (Thrombocytopenia)

10. **Endocrine changes**
    Adrenal insufficiency requiring steroid therapy
    Parathyroid dysfunction resulting in hypercalcemia
    Elevated serum prolactin due to hypothalamic dysfunction

Various Skin Conditions Associated with HIV Infection

1. **Infections and Infestations**

   Viruses
   Herpes simplex & zoster
   Molluscum contagiosum (pox virus)
   Condyloma accumulatum, Verruca vulgaris (papilloma virus)

   Fungal infection
   Candida albicans (thrush)
   Cryptococcus neoformans
   Histoplasma capsulatum

   Protozoan afflictions
   Amebiasis
   Acanthamoeba castellani

   Bacteria and mycobacteria
   Staphylococcus
   Mycobacterium intracellulare & tuberculosis

2. **Malignancies**
   Kaposi's sarcoma
   Hodgkin's disease
   Non-Hodgkin's and Burkitt's lymphoma
   Squamous cell and cloacogenic carcinoma

3. **Miscellaneous**
   Drug eruptions: Sulfonamides and Suramin
   Primary HIV infection
   Seborrheic dermatitis
   Oral "hairy" leukoplakia
   Granuloma annulare-like eruption

Mouth (Oral) manifestations in AIDS Patients

1. **Fungal**
   Candidiasis
   Pseudomembranous
   Atrophic
   Angular cheilitis
   Hyperplastic
   Histoplasmosis
   Geotrichosis
   Cryptococcoses

2. **Bacterial**
   Gingivitis
   Periodontitis
   Necrotizing stomatitis
   Mycobacterium avium intracellulare complex
   Klebsiella stomatitis

3. **Viral**
   Herpes simplex
   Herpes zoster
   Hairy leukoplakia
   Warts

4. **Neoplastic**
   Kaposi's sarcoma
   Non-Hodgkin's lymphoma
   Squamous cell carcinoma

5. **Others**
   Recurrent aphthous ulcers
   Idiopathic thrombocytopenic purpura
   Xerostomia
   Salivary gland enlargement

Nervous system Involvement in AIDS

1. **Infectious complications**

Encephalitis
HIV
Cytomegalovirus
Herpes simplex I, II, & zoster
Adenovirus

Meningitis
HIV
Undetermined
Mycobacterium tuberculosis, avium intracellulare
E. coli
Treponema pallidum
Polymicrobial bacterial infection and others
Fungal
Cryptococcus neoformans
Aspergillus fumigatus
Histoplasma capsulatum
Coccidioides immitis

Brain abscess
Mycobacterium tuberculosis and avium intracellulare, Polymicrobial bacterial infection and others Cryptococcus neoformans, Candida albicans, Toxoplasmosis gondii, Taenia solium (cysticercosis) etc.

Myelopathy
HIV vacuolar myelopathy
Cytomegalovirus
Herpes simplex II & zoster
Epstein-Barr virus
Syphilitic meningomyelitis
Compressive: secondary to epidural abscess

Neuropathy
HIV
Cytomegalovirus
Herpes simplex and post herpetic neuralgia

Myositis
Cause unknown

Progressive multifocal leukoencephalopathy

2. **Brain tumors (Neoplastic)**
Primary tumors
Brain lymphoma
Metastatic disease (including carcinomatous meningitis and compressive myelopathy)
Non-Hodgkin's lymphoma and Hodgkin's
Kaposi's sarcoma
Plasmacytoma

3. **Metabolic disorders**
Drug side effect
Electrolyte abnormality
Vitamin deficiency (Folate, B12, E)

4. **Vascular complications**
Bleeding secondary to immune thrombocytopenia
Subarachnoid & intracerebral hemorrhage
Embolic stroke secondary to endocarditis
Infectious cerebral arteritis (Aspergillus fumigatus)

Hyperthermia by radiat heat, dry sauna, hot tubs, and AUT with or without antimicrobial drugs can eliminate most of these manifestations of AIDS.

How to Avoid AIDS Virus Infection

1. Abstain from sexual intercourse.
2. Have monogamous relationships. If you have been involved in risky behavior during the last 7 years, consider taking the HIV test. "KNOW THY PARTNER"before sex.
3. Condoms: wear condoms during the entire sex act if you do not know your partner.
4. Spermicide: In addition to wearing condoms, use spermicidal foams. The delicate AIDS virus gets killed by spermicide which contain nonoxynol-9. Condoms and spermicides are available in all drug stores.
5. Drug abuse: There are about 1. 2 million intravenous drug users in U. S. A. These addicts should avoid using intravenous drugs. If they have to, they should not share the needle and syringes. Always use sterile needles with disposable syringes.
6. Avoid blood transfusion. If you are undergoing surgery, your own and relatives' blood can be drawn and stored to be used during surgery if needed.
7. An estimated 23% of adult males in U. S. A engage in bisexual activity. The main sexual activity is heterosexual. Nobody dies from not having sex. Use discretion. Love yourself. Millions of Americans get sexually transmitted diseases. Postpone sex if you are not sure of your partner. Look at the reason for saying no to sex. Use common sense. Do not apologize for protecting yourself. Look and search for facts and reasons to say "yes" or "no" to sex. Exert your rights and protect yourself!
8. Observe universal precautions: a. Hand washing before and after patient contact, b. wearing gloves, gowns, protective eye goggles, and masks when there is chance of direct exposure to blood and body fluids, c. proper disposal of needles, intravenous lines, d. wipe the body fluids of patients with absorbing towels and disinfect with 1 in 10 to 100 dilution of 5 % bleach (sodium hypochlorite).
9. Get into dry sauna or hot tubs and practice prophylactic AUT as often as you can if you are in high risk group to eliminate HIV infection.

Who Should Take the HIV Test?

There are many health centers, AIDS centers, and private lab giving this test. They keep this information confidential. It takes up to 24 weeks (usually 6-12 weeks) after infection for antibodies to show in the blood. AIDS is tested on the basis of finding antibodies against the virus. This indicates that someone could be tested negative and still carry the virus. The test method is called ELISA test and many more accurate test are being developed. A new blood test is being developed that can detect the presence of AIDS virus or its components within two days after exposure to the AIDS virus. When this test is available, diagnosis of HIV infection can be made much earlier and more accurately than the ELISA test. The following people should strongly consider getting tested.

1. Any man having sex with another man even once from 1977.
2. Intravenous drugs users by sharing needles and syringes.
3. People from San Francisco, Haiti and Central Africa where the disease is almost epidemic.
4. Prostitutes and their sex mates.
5. Anyone who has not been in a monogamous relationship in the past seven years, who is entering into an intimate relationship, or who is planning marriage and children.
6. Anyone who has symptoms of AIDS (described in this chapter).
7. Patients who have been treated for hemophilia.
8. Those who had blood transfusions between 1977 and March 1985. During this time, blood was not tested for the AIDS virus. You do not get AIDS by giving blood.
9. Had sexual contact with known infected HIV positive person.

The HIV test cannot tell you whether someone has AIDS or AIDS related complex (ARC). The HIV positive test means that the person has been exposed to HIV, has antibodies, and can transmit the virus to others. It is possible to have a false positive test also. That is why positive tests are always checked again. You cannot self diagnose AIDS. Positive test does not mean that you will get AIDS or have AIDS. There is good reason to believe that you will carry the virus all your life. Persons interested in HIV antibody testing should contact their local health department or the AIDS Hotline 1-800-342-2437.

Self Testing for HIV Infection (Home Testing Kits)

AIDS kits are being developed and will be available soon. The kit contains a needle and a blood-absorbing paper. The finger is pricked with the finger stick and the blood is deposited on the special paper. Then it is mailed to the testing laboratories. The result will be mailed back within a few days. The results are kept confidential.

If the HIV Test Positive, What Should be Done Next?

All your efforts should be concentrated on delaying or avoiding AIDS or ARC and to prevent other people from getting it from you. The following measures will help you in that direction:

1. Eat a balanced nutritious diet.
2. Avoid drug and alcoholic abuse. It can damage your immune system.
3. Avoid stress.
4. Get plenty of rest.
5. Keep fit by moderate exercise. Three miles of fast walking daily is the best exercise. Exercise stimulates the immune system also.
6. Have a positive attitude.
7. Contact your physician and have regular checkups.
8. Protect your sex partner by abstaining from sex. If your partner wants to have sex, use condom and spermicidal lubricant containing nonoxynol-9.
9. Inform your other sex partners or those who shared needles with you.
10. Do not share the razors, toothbrush, tweezers, fork, knife, spoons, needles, nail cutter, etc.
11. Do not donate blood or organs for transplant.
12. Clean your blood and semen stains with household ammonia. 1 part in 10 parts of water will kill the AIDS virus.
13. Inform your dentist, health care worker and physician about the HIV positive test.

14. Do not breast feed.
15. Do not bite others and avoid french kissing.
16. Hyperthermia exposure combined with AUT should be undertaken as early as possible.

Change in Life Style if HIV Positive

1. Positive AIDS test does not mean you should change your job. Continue to work.
2. Continue your nonsexual social life.
3. Take care (as described before) to protect others, including sex partners from getting the infection from you.
4. You should tell your sex partners, family members and physician about the HIV test. There is not a single HIV transmitted case reported among those who lived in close family contact with an AIDS patients. There is no need to live in isolation.
5. Continue going to school if you are enrolled.
6. Practice mild to moderate hyperthermia and AUT as recommended. Take care of your physical and psychological health. Moderate exercise like walking cycling are a must for all the patients. All these will affect your immune system and you may never develop the disease.

CHAPTER 17

TREATMENT OF AIDS

If the mountain shiver in cold with what will they wrap them?
If space goes naked with what shall they clothe it?
Allama Prabhu
12th Century Shiva Saint from India

It usually requires a considerable time to determine with certainty the virtues of a new method of treatment and usually takes still longer to ascertain the harmful effects.
Alfred Black

At present, the best way to combat AIDS is to prevent it. A microscopic prevention is better than a mountain of cure. There are no drugs or vaccine available to cure AIDS or prevent AIDS virus infection. AZT (Azydothimidine or Retrovir) is the only drug available at present for treatment. It is not a curative drug. The lay person may ask why there are no effective drugs for AIDS and other viral diseases when there are plenty of antibiotics to end bacterial, fungal and spirochetal infections, and parasitic infestations. Unlike bacteria, AIDS virus and other retroviruses hijack (appropriate) the biosynthetic apparatus of the host cell. Drugs that are effective against the virus will also kill or damage the host cell. This makes it difficult to find a drug or vaccine that will kill the virus and leave the host cell intact. No such drug is on the horizon. The best method is autoimmune urine therapy (AUT), hyperthermia with or without small doses of antimicrobial drugs.

Properties the HIV Antiviral Agent Should Have

1. Effective inhibition of HIV multiplication
2. Least toxic to the organs in the body
3. Should be able to take it orally
4. It should be able to reach the central nervous system
5. It should stay in the body for 30 minutes.
6. Should be inexpensive and easily available.

Only therapy that fits all this criteria is hyperthermia and AUT. Even AZT, the widely used drug for this disease, does not meet all the above criteria. Autoimmune urine therapy and hyperthermia with or without drugs, such as AZT, ddI (in reduced doses) can cure or curtail AIDS.

AZT (Retrovir, Zidovudine, Azydothimidine)

This is the most used, Federal Drug Administration (FDA) approved drug available for AIDS. It is made by Burroughs Wellcome Labs. It is synthesized from herring sperm in a complex chemical process. It blocks the conversion of RNA virus into DNA. It acts by incorporating into a viral enzyme called reverse transcriptase. This enzyme is essential for changing the viral RNA to DNA. It blocks 90% of the detectable HIV multiplication in vitro concentrations of less than 0.13 microgram/ml. It is given orally in doses of 250 mg every four hours. The plasma concentration reaches between 0.16 to 1.46 microgram/ml which is enough to act against HIV. High amounts (75%) of it is absorbed from the intestines. Fourteen percent of it is excreted as AZT unchanged, and 75% of it is as metabolized GAZT in the urine. This is an important finding to remember when we discuss autoimmune urine therapy. About 34 to 84% of AZT is bound to plasma protein. AZT passes the blood brain barrier and enters the brain and the cerebrospinal fluid.

AZT is prescribed for AIDS, cases of advanced ARC with confirmed PCP infection, and T4 lymphocyte count of less than 200 per cubic millimeter of blood. It is given for 24 weeks at doses of about 3 mg/kg body weight every four hours. AZT can cause bone marrow depression, resulting in anemia and low granulocyte white blood cell count. When this occurs, the doses of AZT must be halved or stopped, depending on the severity of the condition. Blood transfusion and vitamin B12 are given. Acetaminophen (Tylenol) increases the toxicity of AZT and should be avoided during AZT therapy. The AZT treatment should be restarted only after the bone marrow shows signs of recovery. AZT therapy is also associated with nausea and vomiting.

AZT improves the quality of life and may prolong life. The cost of the AZT therapy is about $7,500.00 per year, though it costs a fraction to produce it. Most insurance companies pay for therapy. AZT works better with Acyclovir, a drug used in the treatment of herpes. This combination allows the dose of AZT to be reduced to decrease its toxicity. It is used with other unlicensed drugs including dextran. Now AZT given for six weeks for those who are exposed to HIV infection. It is said to suppress the viral multiplication and delay the development of AIDS.

Disadvantages of AZT

1. This drug is very expensive
2. Highly toxic
3. Benefits diminished overtime
4. Does not prevent recurrence or occurrence of PCP
5. Not effective against Kaposi sarcoma.
6. HIV may develop resistance to AZT therapy.

AZT will work better after hyperthermia and AUT. The dose of drug should be reduced. Recent studies show that the drug probenecid prolongs the half life of AZT. This will allow much lower doses of this drug are required. The will lower the cost by half to the patient. Probenecid is a drug given to increase the effect of penicillin by reducing its excretion.

AZT for HIV Infected People without any Symptoms

Recently, the Federal Drug administration has approved AZT use for HIV infected adults who have about 500 /mm3 T4 lymphocytes with no symptoms or early symptoms of AIDS. AZT in these patients will delay the onset of the disease with minimum side effects. For asymptomatic HIV infected patients, the recommended dose is 100 mg every four hours while awake. All symptomatic patients receive 200 mg the first month and then 100 mg every four hours. AUT, hyperthermia with or without small doses of AZT or ddI can eliminate HIV and prevent the development of AIDS.

AZT as Prophylaxis

Risk of HIV infection associated with a single needle stick is estimated to be less than 0.4% (J Infect Dis 1987; 155:558-60). Now the Zidovudine chemoprophylaxis for the health care workers who have been occupationally exposed to HIV has been implemented. It has been reported that giving AZT prophylactically as advertised by the manufacturer may not necessarily prevent HIV infection (N Eng J M:ed 1990,322: 1375-77). The potential benefit of the prophylactic AZT therapy may be offset by its cost and potential (although largely hypothetical) long term complications (J Infect Dis 1989; 160:321-327). AUT and hyperthermia is the best chemoprophylaxis there is.

ddI (2',3'-dideoxyinosine)

ddI is a purine analog. After entering the cell, the drug gets metabolically converted into 2',3'-dideoxyinosine-5'-triphosphate. This active ingredient can remain within the cell for more than 12 hours. ddI suppresses the replication of AIDS virus. It is given orally. Maximum tolerated dose per day is 20 mg per kilogram body weight per day. In preliminary clinical studies, the drug has been tolerated up to 50 weeks. It's major toxic effects are painful peripheral neuropathy and pancreatitis. There are reports of death due to pancreatitis. The other minor complications are: rash, elevated serum liver enzymes and creatine kinase from the muscle,heart beat irregularity due to conduction abnormalities.

This drug causes reduction in serum levels of p24 antigen and increases the T4 lymphocytes. ddI is currently tested in phase II and III clinical trials sponsored by the national institute of allergy and infectious diseases. It is currently made available under an "expanded accesses" program to persons with AIDS and AIDS related complex who are intolerant to AZT or if the latter drug is ineffective (N Eng J Med 1990; 322: 1333-1345).

Antiviral Drugs in the Horizon

At present there are 45 US academic medical centers testing 17 anti-retroviral drugs in 7000 patients in all stages of HIV infection (JAMA, July 28, 1989, vol. 286, p. 452). Autoimmune urine therapy with hyperthermia, as described in Chapter 1, 7, 8, 9, 10 and 18, will act against AIDS virus better than any drug or vaccine presently available.

Dideoxycytidine (Hoffmann-La Roche) and dideoxyadenosine (ddC and ddA): These are nucleoside analogs similar to AZT. They appear to fool HIV into incorporating them into the viruses growing DNA chain during replication. Because analogs lack an important biochemical appendage, the virus cannot finish reproducing its nuclear material and is rendered harmless. In studies with AIDS-infected human cells, ddC stopped viral replication at significantly lower concentrations than AZT says Dr. Broder of NCI. Clinical investigators at NCI are studding ddC in patients with AIDS and AIDS-related complex.

CS-85, CS-87 and CS-91: Developed at Emory University and the University of Georgia. They are closely related to AZT but are less toxic. They have proved effective in hindering the virus's spread in AIDS-infected human cells. Now scientists await results of CS-85 and CS-87 animal tests.

Foscarnet (Sweden's Astra Pharmaceutical Co.): It is in clinical trials in Europe for treatment of cytomegalovirus (a herpes virus) and other herpes infections. It inhibits AIDS virus replication in cultured cells. Astra began tests of Foscarnet among San Francisco AIDS patients with cytomegalovirus retinitis. It causes blindness among AIDS patients.

Ganciclovir (Palo Alto's Syntex Corp.): An analog of acyclovir, is being tested in nationwide clinical trials against cytomegalovirus, and herpes simplex attack of the eyes (retinitis).

D-Penicillamine (Degussa Corp. Teeterboro, NJ): It blocks HIV spread in preliminary clinical trials at George Washington University in Washington, DC. Unfortunately, it also suppressed immune-cell function in some patients. GWU's Dr. David M. Parenti is giving it to AIDS patients every other month. This drug is available in the U.S. by prescription for hepatitis and rheumatoid arthritis.

Alpha-interferon (Hoffman-La Roche, Nutley, NJ) and beta-interferon (Triton Biosciences Inc., Alamed, CA): These are naturally occurring substances in the body. They are mass produced by genetic engineering. Hoffman-La Roche will begin a trial combining alpha-interferon with AZT. New York's Memorial Sloan-Kettering Cancer Center tested alpha-interferon in 16 AIDS patients and found it reduced the lesions of Kaposi's sarcoma in about 30% of patients. According to Dr. Susan Known preliminary evidence suggests it may suppress the growth of the AIDS virus in patients. Initial clinical trials with beta-interferon have shown mixed results according to Dr. William Lang. He is heading studies at Children's Hospital in San Francisco.

Dextran Sulfate: It is not approved for AIDS use. Underground supply is obtained and used by the patient. It is said to work by inhibiting the reverse transcriptase and by preventing the free floating virus from attaching to new T4 lymphocytes.

AL-721: The antiviral properties of this new compound were studied in Weizmann Institute of Israel. It contains 7 parts neutral lipid, 2 parts phosphatidyl choline and 1 part phosphatidyl ethanolamine. This is said to soften the outer shell covering of HIV and preventing it from attaching to T4 lymphocyte receptors thereby preventing infection of T4 lymphocytes.

Ribavirin: This has been used in the past as an antiviral agent against herpes, cytomegalo virus (CMV), flu and colds. It is under study for HIV infection by Dr. Richard B. Roberts of Cornell University. It delays the onset of AIDS.

Peptide T: There is no effective drug or therapy to block entry of HIV into target cells. There are drugs available which block the entry of other types of viruses into the cells. For example amantadine blocks the influenza virus entering mucosal cell lining. My preliminary studies show that instilling or sniffing morning urine into the nose, 2-3 times a day prevent or reduces the incidence of development of influenza and colds. It probably acts by blocking the viral receptors on the nasal mucosal cells to which the cold and influenza virus bind. The National Institute of Mental Health

(NIMH) has synthesized a drug called Peptide T which is believed to prevent the entry of HIV into the cell. Scientists at NIMH (Dr. Peter Bridge) and Karolinska Institute are starting human trials.

CD4 receptors: Biogen Laboratory from Cambridge Massachusetts is commencing human studies with CD4 receptor isolated from the T4 lymphocytes. They attached to free floating viruses and thus prevent them attacking healthy uninfected T4 cells.

GL-223: (Aka compound Q): This drug is derived from a type of Chinese cucumber root. It kills the HIV infected cells. It was used in China to induce abortion. This compound is highly toxic.

Immune System Boosters

Hyperthermia and AUT are better immune boosters than anything we have now.

Diethyldithiocarbamate (DTC, imuthiol): It is supplied by the Merieux Institute in Paris and Miami. It stimulates the hormone Hepatosin production in liver. Hepatosin stimulates production and maturation of T4 cells. Thus it halts the progression of AIDS-related complex (ARC) to AIDS, according to M.D. Anderson Hospital in Houston. Merieux reports similar results in France. Studies are in progress at six centers in the U.S., according to American Health, (June, 1987). As this substance is not available, many AIDS patients use antabuse which has the same effect. Antabuse is used in alcohol addiction treatment. If you are taking either one of these drugs, do not drink alcohol.

Imreg (Imreg Inc., New Orleans): It raised immune responses in 15 of 29 patients in a preliminary study, says Dr. A. Arthur Gottlieb, president of Imreg. Full clinical trials have been started for 150 patients with AIDS or ARC. Imreg's Dr. Clifford Kern reports no toxicity in over 100 patients treated.

Thymostimulin (Serono Laboratories of Randolph, MA): It is being tested on ARC patients in four U.S. hospitals.

Granulocyte Monocyte-Colony Stimulating Factor (GM-CSF) (Cambridge's Genetics Institute): It is an immune system booster. It increases white cells. GM-CSF is tested with AIDS patients at New England Deaconess Hospital and UCLA. Sandoz Pharmaceuticals of East Hannover, NJ, is sponsoring the trials.

Azimexon (Boehringer Mannheim): It boost immune system function in some ARC patients. Safety trials are conducted at the Institute for Immunological Disorders in Houston.

Thymopentin (TP5) (Ortho Pharmaceutical Corp. of Raritan, NJ): It is under study with combination treatment with ribavirin by Dr. Michael J. Scolaro and colleagues at St. Vincent Medical Center in Los Angeles on AIDS patients with Kaposi's sarcoma and secondary infections.

Interlukin-II: Discussed by Dr. Robert Gallo and his co-workers may have some benefit. The problem with his protein is that it stimulates both immune system and AIDS viral multiplication.

Isoprinosine: It stimulate certain functions of the immune system including the T4 cell production. This drug is used in combination with Ribavirin by some AIDS patients.

Typhoid Vaccine: This vaccine has been patented (N0. 4711876 in Dec.8,1987) for use in AIDS by Salavatore Catapano, 72 years old and a medical technologist in the Navy. He claims the disappearance of mental and respiratory symptoms in AIDS patients. It may not work for everybody. It is given in the form of two injections(0.75 to 1.00 ml. marketed by Wyeth lab.) a week, then once a week, then once a month. He advises not to combine with other drugs such as AZT or radiation. He is convinced that AIDS is really syphilis and believes that using AZT is like passing death sentence. He claims that after 15 shots of Typhoid vaccine, AIDS patients who were negative for syphilis became positive (Spin Nov. 1988). The Typhoid vaccine acts as a nonspecific stimulator of the immune system.

Naltrexone: is used in the treatment of opium and heroin addiction. It is a narcotic antagonist. It increases the endorphin levels. This increases the sensitivity of the receptor sites on immune system cells. AIDS patients show high levels of natural alpha interferon. Administration of this drug reduces alpha interferon levels by making it bind to immune system cells.

AUT and hyperthermia gives better results than most of these drugs. American Foundation for AIDS Research (40 West 57th Street, Suite 406, New York, N.Y. 10019, 212-333-3118) has published "AIDS/HIV Experimental Treatment Directory" (1988). General readers are referred to this directory.

Immune Therapeutic Agents Available or being Tried

1. Hormones from the thymus gland (thymosin fraction V, thymostimulin, TP-1, thymopentin,thymic humoral factor)
2. Lymphokines (interleukin-2, tumor necrosis factor)
3. Interferon (alpha, gamma)
4. Immune Stimulating Agents (inosine,imuthiol)
5. Hematologic Growth Factors (GM-CSF)

Autoimmune urine therapy combined with hyperthermia is the best immune therapeutic agent available. This therapy will stimulate all the above immune system factors and will help to cure or curtail HIV infection and AIDS.

Opportunistic Infection in AIDS, Clinical Syndromes and Available Therapy (PO=Oral intake, IV=Given through the vein, IM=given through the muscle)

Protozoa

1. Pneumocystis carinii: causes pneumonia; treated with trimethoprim-sulfamethoxalole (TMP-SMZ), pentamidine isothionate, Dapsone (IV, IM, or aerosol)
2. Toxoplasma gondii: causes encephalitis, brain abscess; treated with sulfadiazine, pyrimethamine and folinic acid (PO)
3. Cryptosporidium muris: causes gastroenteritis, treated with spiramycin (PO)
4. Isospora belli: causes gastroenteritis, treated with TMP-SMZ (PO)

Fungi

1. Candida albicans: causes oropharyngitis, treated with nystatin suspension (PO) or clotrimazole troches; esophagitis by ketoconazole (PO) or amphotericin B (IV)

2. Cryptococcus neoformans: causes meningitis, pneumonia, fungemia; treated with amphotericin B (IV) or amphotericin B (IV) along with flucytosine (IV)

Virus

1. Cytomegalovirus (CMV): causes chorioretinitis, pneumonia, hepatitis, colitis, disseminated infection, adrenalitis; treated with DHP [9-(1,3-dihydroxy 2-propoxymethyl) guanine] (IV)
2. Herpes simplex: produces mucocutaneous lesions (perineal and oral); treated with acyclovir (PO or IV)
3. Varicella-zoster: primary varicella infection, local or disseminated herpes zoster; treated with acyclovir (PO orIV)
4. Epstein-Barr virus: causes oral hairy leukoplakia, lymphoid interstitial pneumonitis, B-cell lymphoma; at present no treatment is available

Mycobacteria

1. M. avium intracellular: causes gastroenteritis, disseminated infection (blood, liver, spleen,marrow, lungs, etc.) ; treated with isoniazid, rifamide, clofazimine and ethambutol combinations.

The best therapy for all these opportunistic infections is to practice AUT, hyperthermia, with or without small doses of specific anti microbial, anti parasitic drugs.

AIDS Vaccine

There are several vaccines ready to be tested. They are made of the virus cell membrane part of the HIV virus. The Salk Institute has developed a vaccine based on the inactivated whole virus. The Salk's AIDS vaccine cleared the viruses from the blood in two out of three chimpanzees and protected them against reinfection for nine months. Nineteen men suffering from AIDS related complex received this vaccine. They showed improvement in ARC. 60% of them showed an increased skin sensitivity and enhanced immunity. A vaccine known as GP-160 made from the HIV outer coat shows promising results. This vaccine is being tested by Dr. Clifford Lane of the National Institute of Allergy and Infectious Disease. The vaccine may prevent healthy people from becoming infected with AIDS virus. It is tested on 120 volunteers.

Recently Paul Naylor and Allen L. Goldstein of George Washington University identified another HIV protein, P17. It stimulates production of antibodies. The Food and Drug Administration has approved trials. George J. Todaro has produced a vaccine from two proteins from the exterior wall of the AIDS virus. Dr. William Jarret of University of Glasgow Veterinary School is studying immune stimulating complexes called Iscoms. More than 25 research projects by Drug Companies and Research Institutes are doing research to come up with a vaccine (Science Vol. 259,N0.4 P126). Any vaccine developed should have three prong attack on the AIDS virus.

1. Should produce antibodies to attack the free floating newly released viruses.
2. Should be able to protect the vaccinated individual against infection with AIDS virus(like smallpox and polio vaccines).
3. Vaccine should be able to attack and eliminate virus infected cells without harming other healthy cells of similar type.

AUT along with hyperthermia is the best vaccine any one can have. Give it a chance to work.

Cost for the AIDS Patients and Liability

The medical expenses, suffering and loss of life due to AIDS is staggering. Women patients with AIDS die faster than men. For example in New York, 1,000 women with this disease lived less than two years compared to 10,000 men who made it past 2-1/2 years. The possible explanation given is that these women were poor, sickly, drug users and did not get good care. Up to 25- 50% of those persons who are HIV positive will develop the disease. The U.S. government has spent billions of dollars on research and education. The average lifetime hospital cost per AIDS patient is $147,000. According to Rand corporation, treating AIDS patient will cost $37 billion by mid 1991 and could reach $113 billion. Most AIDS patients are between the ages of 20 - 40. The indirect cost including loss of earnings due to sickness or death are estimated to be $36 billion by 1991. Life and health insurance companies refuse insurance coverage for HIV positive individuals. The Canadian subsidiary of the Prudential Insurance Company is advancing part of its life insurance to AIDS patients to spend on their care. I hope this method of prepayment is adopted in the U.S.

The other side of AIDS is to collect money on the basis of fear, relationship and malpractice. The famous case is that of actor Rock Hudson and his lover. The jury awarded $22 million dollars to compensate for the fear of acquiring AIDS to the homosexual lover of the actor even though he was tested negative for AIDS virus. The latest case is that of 5 year old Alex Edwards and his parents who were awarded 28.7 million dollars in Arizona for transfusing blood and plasma when the baby was two days old and infecting it with AIDS. The unfortunate physician who transfused the blood to the save the life is a neonatologist named Abraham Kuruvilla. Alex tested positive in December 1986 (AMA news June 29,1990). To me both the awards are outrageous and money cannot buy life except a mercedes or a Rolls Royce and a huge diamond ring to the plaintiff's attorney. There are private agencies who buy the life insurance policies of AIDS patients at reduced face value and advance the money.

AIDS Promoters

There are many advertisements all over the country guaranteeing the AIDS cure. They vary widely and range from injection of hydrogen peroxide and typhoid vaccine to ingesting large quantities of lead and snake venom. The sellers claim them as miracle cures. These products cost from $10.00 to $200.00. For example, there is a four page pamphlet selling for $13.50 titled Exciting Miracle Breakthrough. All it tells is a four page description of AIDS and safe sex. Another product comes from AZT Laboratories costing $200.00. It has nothing to do with AZT drug used in AIDS. A company called Bottled Marrow Tech, Inc. advertised that it will remove healthy bone marrow and keep it preserved (by deep freezing). It is to be used if such a person develops AIDS later. The cost is enormous and we don't even know whether such a deep frozen bone marrow can be used with any benefit in AIDS. There was an institute called USHA Institute which claimed it cured AIDS. It is shut down now.

There are products claimed to stimulate the immune system. As they are advertised for cancer patients, these products are nothing but high potency vitamins and minerals. One can buy these at health food stores for a fraction of the cost. People sell Sani-Phone protective mouth pieces for telephones to prevent the spread of AIDS. Business entrepreneurs and con people always try to exploit when there is fear and ignorance.

To find out about a particular cure, call the Communicable Disease Center or Atlanta National AIDS hot lines (1-800-342-2437), for gay and bisexuals (1-800-221-7044) or Amfair (212-719-0033).

Final Preparation

Once the patient knows about the HIV diagnosis, gently encourage the person to examine and assess the important issues and priories. The patient should decide what he/she wants to do with the time left. It is like any other terminal disease. Clear all the unfinished business. In order to avoid future difficulties, select a family member or trusted friend to carry out your wishes. Assign legal power of attorney to such a person. Prepare a living will. Discuss all the issues of your property, insurance, and end stage care (i.e. prolong the life by artificial respiration, and other heroic measures if the ailing person is not capable of proper judgement). As the disease progresses, the brain gets affected. So any legal decision made in later stages of AIDS can be questioned. Do not consider suicide. Focus on hope for prolonging the life with autoimmune urine therapy and other combination of medications. Plan your life. Death is a terminal illness. When it comes, we do not know. Enjoy your life what may come. My final advice is to try AUT and hyperthermia before you think death.

IF YOU TRY WHAT I RECOMMEND IN THIS BOOK, THERE IS NO REASON TO HAVE FINAL PREPARATIONS FULFILLED

CHAPTER 18

AUTOIMMUNE URINE THERAPY (AUT), HYPERTHERMIA AND DRUGS FOR HIV POSITIVE INDIVIDUALS AND AIDS PATIENTS

How To Cure or Curtail AIDS

For extreme diseases, extreme methods of cure
Hippocrates

If I have a thousand ideas a year and only one turns good, I am satisfied.
Alfred Nobel

Those who refuse to go beyond facts rarely get as far as fact.
T. H. Huxley

Chances favor only the prepared mind.
Louis Pasteur

How Does Autoimmune Urine Therapy Combined with Hyperthermia and Drugs Work Against HIV and AIDS?

I do not know of any drug for any disease that has such a multi-prong attack on a disease as the urine has. **Urine is the best antibiotic, antiparasitic, antitoxic, antianemic, anticancer, antiviral, antibacterial, antifungal, immune system stimulating,**

health-building, anti-aging, cost-free product ever manufactured. The following are ways how autoimmune urine therapy combined with hyperthermia and antiviral drugs work to cure or curtail AIDS and eliminate the AIDS virus from our body (See Figs. 1-13).

Many of the explanation given how hyperthermia and autoimmune urine therapy acts on the AIDS virus also applies to all the causative agents of opportunistic infection, leprosy, tuberculosis, rabies and any other incurable, chronic debilitating diseases. Autoimmune urine therapy with hyperthermia and drugs have a better chance of eliminating AIDS virus, opportunistic infection and many other diseases as described in this book.

Even if one of the explanation, reasoning, and method I give in this book proves right in treating any disease discussed in this book or any other disease mentioned or not mentioned in this book I am satisfied.

1. **Autoimmune urine therapy with hyperthermia and drugs Prevents the AIDS virus from attaching to the lymphocytes receptor sites:** Autoimmune urine therapy (AUT) and Hyperthermia may act on T_4 (CD4) receptors on lymphocytes. It prevents the circulating viral particles in the blood from infecting the healthy T_4 lymphocytes. This increases the number of healthy T4 cells and brings the ratio of T4/T8 to more than one. This ratio drops to 0.5 or less in AIDS patients. When this happens, the liberated virions are unable to impair the "immune system activation." This allows the T4, T8, B cells, plasma cells and macrophages to perform their function as discussed before.

For AIDS to develop, the viruses must gain access to the circulation of the potential host. Here, the HIV with the help of a surface antigen called GP 120 attaches to the T4 cells surface antigen (CD4). Experimentally (in vitro) such receptor sites can be blocked by monoclonal antibodies. They prevent HIV from getting attached to receptors on the lymphocytes. If the virus is unable to bind to the T4 cells, it cannot start infection. Thus, urine and hyperthermia therapy can be a effective as a prophylactic and curative therapy against AIDS virus infection.

2. Inhibits enzyme reverse transcriptase (Fig. 11): Once inside the cell, the HIV viral RNA, with the help of the enzyme reverse transcriptase, copies its RNA into DNA. This converted viral DNA enters the nucleus and integrates itself into the genome (host gene, DNA) of the host cell. Here the virus may remain dormant without dividing in the host cells (provirus). Autoimmune urine therapy and hyperthermia inhibits the enzyme reverse transcriptase and its associated changes. There is a possibility that AUT prevents or inhibits the RNA virus from changing into DNA. Without such a change, the virus will not be able to reproduce, thus ending the infection. Many drugs such as Suramin, HPA 23, Foscarnet, AZT, ddI, Rifabutin, and Ribavirin, as well as **hyperthermia, acts by inhibiting or inactivating the reverse transcriptase enzyme**. AUT is probably as effective as these drugs and has no toxic side-effects on the body and it is free. Hyperthermia and AUT will enhance the effect of these drugs.

3. Prevents viral DNA from entering the host nucleus: Once the virus changes its RNA to DNA, it has to enter the host nucleus. Without such an entry, the DNA cannot be incorporated into the cell nucleus. AUT, with hyperthermia, inhibits or delays the entry of viral DNA into host cell's nucleus. This will prevent or slowdown genome development and viral incorporation inside the cell nucleus.

4. Prevents HIV multiplication induction by foreign proteins: The white cells are stimulated by foreign antigens to divide. Due to this stimulation, the T4 cell produces interlukin-II, which further promotes T cell growth and division. The virus also multiplies inside the T4 cell. These multiplied viruses kill the cell as the viral particles are released. These viruses in turn attach to new T4 cells. This cycle repeats itself and results in depletion of T4 cells. At a critical point, the impaired immune response results. Autoimmune urine therapy prevents T4 cell depletion by preventing the new virus from attacking the newly-formed T4 cells. AUT drastically reduces the foreign protein stimulated T4 cell division. During AUT, hyperthermia and fasting, no foreign proteins are introduced. The existing foreign proteins and cofactors are used and eliminated. The viral multiplication also slows down due to lack of foreign protein stimulated T4 cell division. With continued AUT, hyperthermia and fasting, the total body viral pool is gradually depleted. This results in a bouncing back of the immune system, which attacks the AIDS virus.

5. **Prevents HIV expression:** The work of virologists such as Gallo at NCI and W. Hazeltine and M. Essex at Harvard has shown that the AIDS virus has as many as nine genes. T cell activation and viral expression are linked to viral genes. Autoimmune urine therapy plays an important role in promoting the immune system activation (T cells) without viral replication (expression) by suppressing the viral genes. Hyperthermia eliminates may of the free circulating AIDS virus. The lymphocyte production is enhanced. Many of the infected T cells are destroyed due to hyperthermia and come out in urine. Urine during and after hyperthermia is loaded with antigens and basic building material for lymphocyte and antibody production.

6. **Antibody development to genetically different mutated AIDS virus:** Once activated, HIV reproduces rapidly and acts carelessly, resulting in variable HIV genome. This makes it difficult for the immune system to react due to lack or delay in recognition of specific changed viral antigens. This has made the development of the vaccine especially challenging. Continuous autoimmune urine therapy along with multiple hyperthermia exposure produces antibodies to many genetically different HIV. Thus, the antibodies act on the virus no matter what change it has undergone. In this way autoimmune urine therapy and hyperthermia is more effective in wiping out genetically different HIV infections.

7. **Stimulation of B and T cells to perform their Function (Fig. 6, 12):** Urine contains AIDS virus, their degraded broken down components and lymphokines (interlukin-II, interferon, etc.). When urine is taken orally, these components are denatured by digestive juices. These antigenic viral substances and lymphokines gets

absorbed into the blood and lymph stream. The viral particles, or part of it are eaten by macrophages which produce interlukin-1, which in turn activates the T cells system. Other foreign antigens also stimulate T cells and B cells. The T cells produce lymphokines and along with urine lymphokines, stimulate T and B cells. One such lymphokine is interlukin-II. It is a potent stimulator of T cell growth and differentiation. Another lymphokine called alpha interferon is absorbed from the urine (produced by T4 cells) and stimulates macrophage and natural killer cells (line of T8 cytotoxic cells). Broken down lymphokines from urine act as building blocks to produce more lymphokines. Thus, urine, with its hundreds of biochemical (bodies own proteins, lymphokines, broken down cells and viral particles, etc.), activates macrophages, natural killer cells, antibody-producing B cells, cytotoxic T8 cells and lymphokine production. Hyperthermia increases the out put of lymhphokines and with AUT stimulates or enhances the effects of immune defense system. This helps to create an effective immune defense against invading and invaded AIDS viruses, opportunistic infections and cancers.

T4 helper cells play the primary role in the overall modulation of the immune system response. These cells act by secreting lymphokines, recognizing foreign antigen, proliferation of T cells colony, and making B cells to produce specific antibodies and modulate cytotoxic suppressor activity of T8 cells. Depletion of T4 cells has a devastating effect on the immune defense system and exposes the body to many opportunistic infections and cancers. Every day thousands of immune defense cells (T and B cells) are killed in the AIDS battle. Many components of these killed cells are passed in the urine. By practicing AUT and hyperthermia, these are fed back into the body. They act as potent stimulators of T and B cell production and increase their fighting capacity against AIDS. AUT, with its multiple pharmacological compounds and hyperthermia prevent the release of viral particles from infected cells. It prevent the liberated HIV from attaching to T4 cell receptor sites. The AIDS antibodies produced by autoimmune urine therapy neutralize any free floating AIDS viruses. By these processes, the number of T4 cells attacked by the virus is diminished and T4 cell population is increased.

8. **Production of T and Tn antibodies which prevent AIDS virus attachment to Host Cells:** The AIDS patient's urine probably contains substances similar to T and Tn antigen seen in cancer patients. Hyperthermia enhances the release of these antigens and similar substances. When we drink our own urine rich in T and Tn antigens, it is absorbed in the gut, resulting in antibody synthesis for T and Tn type antigens. These antibodies prevent the attachment of the AIDS virus to the T4 cell and macrophage surface antigen. This results in the prevention of reinfection of healthy T cells, monocytes, macrophage, stem cells in bone marrow, and other susceptible cells. It also prevents cell-to-cell transmission of viruses and cell-to-cell adhesion (syncytia) induced T cell death. This will result in a normal immune system with its fighting capacity. These antibodies will prevent sticking of one lymphocyte to others, which is responsible for the rapid depletion of the T4 lymphocytes and AIDS.

9. **Antibody production against the mutated virus:** The entire gut wall (lamina propria) is lined with billions of antibody-producing plasma cells. By drinking all the urine, along with fasting and hyperthermia, these broken down viral products in the urine are absorbed through the gut wall. Hyperthermia enhances the absorption of antigens from the gut. They are presented to plasma cells along with the other immune defense cells in the gut wall. They in turn manufacture antibodies against the different components of HIV. No matter how much the HIV mutates, the plasma cells continue to produce antibodies against mutated HIV and its parts. These antibodies attack the HIV antigens and neutralize these viruses, as they are released. **AUT and hyperthermia is the best vaccine there is.**

10. Prevention of reproduced virus seeds from being released from the cell nucleus: The AIDS virus, once produced inside the host cell genetic material (nucleus) has to break off from the main protein chain to produce viral particles. It is like pearls breaking of from the pearl string. The enzyme nuclease plays a role in snipping off HIV from the chain of virion produced inside the T4 lymphocytes. AUT and hyperthermia inhibits enzyme nuclease activity. This reduces or prevents the release of multiplying virion from the cell nucleus. The virus multiplies but cannot separate from the main chain to come out of the cell nucleus. It is trapped like an insect in a spider web. This leads to a reduction in the number of viral particles circulating and infecting new T4 cells. This will result in an increased number of new T4 cells and enhances the immune defense system.

11. Enhancing the virus exposure to the Immune system and the sugar coating acting as food for hungry cells (Fig. 6, 9):

The AIDS virus envelope is heavily sugar-coated, according to William Hazeltine from Harvard's Dana Farber Cancer Institute in Boston. That is why the antibodies in our body cannot see the viral parts inside the sugar coat to mount an attack. It is like a turtle within a turtle shell. During autoimmune urine therapy and hyperthermia, along with fasting, no sugars are eaten. Total body sugars are used up. The sugar level on all the cells, as well as in the viral particles, also drops. So the body cells have to meet its glucose needs from within. Thus, these viruses, which are tiny and sugar-coated, can be used as food by sugar starved body cells. The fats from fat cells and its breakdown products (ketone bodies) coat the AIDS viruses. Now the viruses are like butter-coated, syrup-drenched pancakes. The body cells swallow them as food materials. This results in elimination of free floating viruses in the body by the non-immune defense cells.

As the sugar content of the viral coat is reduced (depletion of body sugars due to fasting and hyperthermia), the true identity of the virus and its parts are recognized by the immune system. This makes it easier for the antibodies to attack the viruses. That is why it is important to fast during autoimmune urine therapy. During hyperthermia, the virus shell is softened. This will prevent it from attaching to receptors and infecting new cells. Further, the cell wall of the virus is weakened. This will make it easier to identify and attack the virus by immune system.

12. Multiple type of virus antibody production: Most viruses have three genes. The AIDS virus has nine genes identified so far. This is a weak point in the invader. It comes out in urine broken down into its multiple gene parts. These are further broken down denatured by hyperthermia, the stomach and intestinal juices. These viral parts are absorbed and act as antigens. Thus many different kinds of antibodies are produced due to stimulation by multiple antigens. During hyperthermia, these antigens output is enhanced. This will result in enhanced antibody production. These antibodies act against the AIDS virus, attacking its various genetic parts. The same processes takes place with other infections.

13. Viral gp 120 neutralization by vasoactive intestinal polypeptide (VIP) (Fig. 11): The outer cell wall gp 120 glycoprotein of AIDS virus, without any other parts of the virus, can bind and kill cultured mouse brain nerve cells (Douglas E. Brenneman et al, Nature, Oct. 13, 1988). This study found that a hormone called vasoactive intestinal polypeptide (VIP) shares many of the same genetic sequences found in gp 120. It can prevent nerve cell death by blocking gp 120 from binding to nerve cells in tissue culture. Unfortunately, VIP in the human body would not cross the blood brain barrier to enter the nervous system. Fortunately, VIP is produced in the brain also. By practicing autoimmune urine therapy and hyperthermia, the VIP produced in the intestine is absorbed into the circulation in large qualities. Due to fasting during autoimmune urine therapy, none of it is lost in the feces. Usually massive amounts of digestive enzymes, along with VIP, are poured into the gut to mix with food and finally evacuated in feces.

During autoimmune urine therapy, fasting and hyperthermia, the amount of VIP content in the gut increases many fold. Its activity is also enhanced by hyperthermia. It is easily absorbed along with the urine and water we drink. It will combine with the circulating gp

120 of the viral envelope. Thus it prevents gp 120 from being attached to nerve cells located outside the brain and spinal cord. This prevents any HIV attack on the peripheral neurons, especially those belonging to the autonomic nervous system.

Further, autoimmune urine therapy and hyperthermia enhances the output of VIP in the brain. This reduces the chances of gp 120 attacking the brain and spinal cord. During hyperthermia, the blood brain barrier is broken. This will allow VIP from the blood to enter the brain and attack gp 120 and eliminate it's lethal effects on the brain. Due to fasting and hyperthermia associated with autoimmune urine therapy, VIP-like molecules (peptide-T) are produced. They can enter the brain easily and block the lethal effects of gp 120 on the brain cells. Thus autoimmune urine therapy effectively prevents and alleviates the brain damage caused by the AIDS virus. AUT and hyperthermia can block all the AIDS afflictions of the central and peripheral nervous system.

14. Effects of increased VIP in preventing diarrhea (Fig. 7): AIDS-associated diarrhea and other gastrointestinal afflictions are blamed on emaciation and intestinal infection. The circulating gp 120 from HIV can also attack nerve cells located in Meissner's and Auerbach's plexuses in the intestinal wall. This will result in deranged functioning. This will upset the intestinal movement, and change digestion, absorption, and production of digestive enzymes and hormones. Autoimmune urine therapy with hyperthermia, by reducing the loss of vasoactive intestinal peptide and increasing its production, increases the body levels of VIP. VIP will prevent binding of the gp 120 part of AIDS virus with the nerve cells (of Meissner and Auerbach plexus) in the gut wall. This process is enhanced by hyperthermia. This maintains proper functioning of the digestive organ. It will control diarrhea, increase absorption, end malnutrition and maintain harmony.

15. Increased production of hepatosin: Fasting will give complete rest to all the digestive organs, including the liver and pancreas. When this is followed by autoimmune urine therapy and hyperthermia, it results in increased production of a liver hormone called hepatosin. It is similar to the hormone thymosin from the thymus gland. It regulates T lymphocytes after birth. This hormone speeds up maturation of T4 cells, improves T4/T8 ratio, and increases lymphocyte killer cells response. Imuthiol (DTC) is a complex chemical said to act in the same fashion. Without using toxic drugs, you can achieve the same results by autoimmune urine therapy and hyperthermia.

16. AUT act as a monoclonal antibody: Vaccines need to be developed to prevent HIV from binding to target cells. Vaccines will produce antibodies, which will bind with free floating viruses or will act on the receptors on cells, thus preventing the virus from entering the cells. Viruses cannot survive outside the cell, because viruses are true parasites. There are several vaccines which have been developed and tested. Vaccines work by producing antibodies against the HIV. Unfortunately this disease develops in the presence of neutralizing antibodies to HIV. So we do not know how effective vaccines will be. Vaccines in the form of monoclonal antibodies can be effective. AUT is as good a vaccine and monoclonal antibody anyone can get against all infectious diseases, including AIDS. The AIDS antibodies coming out of urine, with the help of hyperthermia, gastric and intestinal secretions, and proteins from cells within our body form monoclonal antibody like substances. They specifically act on the AIDS virus and virus infected cells, opportunistic infections and cancer cells.

17. Softening of viral membrane, which will prevent attachment to the host cells (Fig. 13): AL-721, a lipid compound, is being studied in the Weizman Institute for AIDS. It acts at the stage of viral binding to target cells. There are many AIDS patients who make compounds similar to AL-721 in home brew or makeshift factories using soybean and egg yolk lecithin. Many health food stores carry egg lecithin (eggscat) of poor quality. It acts by softening the viral and host target cell membrane. The virus has a rigid cell membrane as do the receptor sites on the host cells. By softening these membranes, HIV is unable to align and bind to receptor site of T4 cells. Al-721 contains 7 parts neutral lipids, 2 parts phosphatidyl choline and 1 part phosphatidyl ethanolamine. It is taken orally 20-30 grams a day.

Autoimmune urine therapy and hyperthermia does a better job than AL-721 or any other related compounds. While undergoing AUT and hyperthermia, the person undergoes fasting for four to twelve weeks, depending on the patient's condition. During fasting, the body uses stored glucose the first day. Then it begins to breakdown body fat stores for energy. Thus, lipid content and it derivatives (ketone bodies) in the blood serum increases. These endogenous body lipids and ketone bodies soften the outer viral wall and the host cells. During fasting, the body fats are extracted from the fat cells by the enzyme lipase. The lipase levels also go up due to heightened fat breakdown (lipolysis) and hyperthermia. The lipase also starts acting on the hard shell casing of the AIDS virus. Same thing happens during hyperthermia. These lipids and lipase alter the structure of the viruses. This will prevent the reinfection of T4 cells by newly released viral particles. The antibodies recognize these weakened viruses and attack them.

Urine contains urea, a nonprotein nitrogen (NPN), creatinine, etc., (see Chapter 7). When urine is ingested, blood level of these compounds are raised immediately. These compounds soften and alter the surface of the viral covering. These compounds also change the outer cell wall of the host cell to a level that will not allow the virus to bind to receptors of T4 cells. Even if they bind to T4 cells, the binding is not firm enough to allow the virus to enter the T4 cell interior. Thus, AUT is effective against AIDS and HIV positive people.

Massaging the body skin with urine and hyperthermia also plays an important role. Lipids are forced into circulation by fasting, urine massaging and hyperthermia from the skin fat. They coat and soften the virus and host cell membrane. The viruses are unable to bind to T4 cells and infect them. Urine, along with its lipid, also acts on Langerhans cells in skin which contain the AIDS virus. They free them of AIDS virus infection.

18. Fasting, hyperthermia and AUT produces an environment in which the AIDS virus cannot thrive: Fasting, hyperthermia along with autoimmune urine therapy, will change the fluid media in which T4 cells and viruses are floating. In this altered media HIV will be unable to bind effectively to the T4 receptors. Thus, reinfection of T4 cells does not take place. Lipids and various peptides liberated into circulation during hyperthermia, fasting and urine drinking create many receptor-like locus to which the liberated virus bind. Once the HIV binds to these free-floating molecules which act on "decoy receptors," the HIV will lose ability to bind to any other cells, including T4 cells. Thus, the reinfection of the T4 cells is virtually eliminated.

19. Production of T4 Antibodies which occupy T4 receptors and prevent viral attachment to these cells (Fig. 13): Urine contains part of T4 receptor protein to which the AIDS virus binds. During hyperthermia many lymphocytes are destroyed. This results in release of millions CD4 receptors into the urine. These receptors are absorbed from the intestines. T and B lymphocytes produce antibodies, interferons, lymphokines which act against T4 receptor sites (against CD4 receptor site). Thus there are no more receptor sites left on the T4 cells for HIV to attach and enter these cells. Further, the AUT and hyperthermia increases the level of free floating CD4 receptors. Any released new viruses will bind to these free floating CD4 receptors. Many healthy T4 cells are left intact without being invaded by the AIDS virus. The immune system remains intact and recovers.

20. Production of lymphokine activated cells which kills AIDS Virus: Dr. Steven Rosenberg, (National Cancer Institute of Bethesda, MD USA), in a novel experiment achieved complete remission of some tumors (especially kidney tumors). He took white blood cells from the cancer patient's blood and incubated them in the laboratory with Interlukin-II. The latter is involved in the stimulation of immune systems cells. These cells are called LAK cells short for lymphokine activated cells. They are injected back into the patient, along with Interlukin-II. About 13% of his patients obtained complete remission. The problem with this therapy is patients become extremely sick and develop heart failure and low blood pressure. This treatment is expensive and life threatening. Autoimmune urine therapy and hyperthermia serves the same purpose as the above experimental therapy. By feeding back the urine as in total autoimmune urine therapy and hyperthermia, the Interlukin-II levels go up. It comes in contact with healthy killer T8 lymphocytes and is converted into LAK cells. These LAK-like cells start attacking the virus infected cells and eat them. This process takes time to develop with autoimmune urine therapy. It costs nothing and is not life threatening.

21. Increases the production of HIV activated lymphocyte killer cells: Dr. Steve Rosenberg has modified the above LAK treatment. He obtains the leukocytes that are assigned to the tumors (tumor infiltrating white cells). These cells are grown in tissue culture into billions of cells with the help of Interlukin-II. Bits of tumor pieces are also fed to these multiplying cells. Within a few weeks, these cells are injected back into the patients circulation. They will home back to the cancer site and start attacking them. These cells are 50 to 100 times more effective in killing tumors. These primed tumor infiltrating cells are specific for only that particular type tumor from which they originated. These cells swarm the tumor like termites attacking dead wood, nibbling it away.

In autoimmune urine therapy and hyperthermia the same phenomenon takes place. The AIDS virus does undergo degradation in the body and is excreted in the urine. This processes is enhanced by the hyperthermia. This urine is taken orally. These viruses and their parts are like inactivated bacteria and viral vaccines (killed by heat or formalin, or attenuated) used in different vaccines. They are absorbed by the gastrointestinal tract where they are presented to killer T4 cells, as well as to other immune cells. These cells become VACK, short for "virus activated cell killers." These VACK cells, with the help of Interlukin-II from the body start multiplying in millions. Bits and pieces of AIDS virus are presented to them from autoimmune urine therapy continuously. The AIDS viruses they engulf remind them of their primary mission. That is, then seek and destroy the AIDS virus and infected cells within the body. Thus, autoimmune urine therapy helps to eliminate the AIDS virus infection, AIDS, cancer and many other diseases.

22. Autoimmune urine therapy and hyperthermia prevents infected T4 lymphocytes killing healthy T4 cells: The viral glycoprotein displayed on the HIV infected T4 cell binds with uninfected T4 cells and fuse with it. This results in formation of syncytial cell. According to the studies, by this phenomenon, one infected cell can kill up to 500 uninfected T4 cells. This phenomenon helps to explain how massive T4 cell destruction takes place in HIV infected people. By practicing autoimmune urine therapy with hyperthermia, various components in urine prevent the attachment of infected T4 cells with healthy T4 cells. Further during autoimmune urine therapy the plasma cells will manufacture anti HIV envelope antibodies. These antibodies attach to the infected T4 cells and prevent them sticking to healthy T4 cells, thus preventing the massive destruction of healthy T4 cells by clumping. Hyperthermia destroys many infected T4 cells and removes it from circulation. This therapy prevents the massive depletion of T4 cells and brings an end to the progression of HIV infection into full blown AIDS.
Hyperthermia also kills the mycoplasma (cofactor) infected red blood cells which are said to destroy lymphocytes and help in development of AIDS. AUT produces antibodies against the mycoplasma bacteria. Combining AUT with hyperthermia can reduce or prevent the destruction of lymphocytes which are essential for the proper functioning of the immune system.

23. Produces anti HIV envelope antibodies which mark the infected cells to be dealt by immune system: By practicing autoimmune urine therapy and hyperthermia, there is increased production of anti-HIV envelope antibodies. These attach to the cells infected with HIV. Thus, they are marked to be destroyed by specific host effector cells (JAMA, 1989, vol. 261, p. 3002).

24. Increases the lymphokines which suppress viral multiplication: The T4 cells of the AIDS patient produce lymphokine. They suppress the virus replication in infected cells. During autoimmune urine therapy and hyperthermia, the lymphokines that are leaking through urine are ingested. They are absorbed from the gut and circulate all over the body where they suppress the multiplication of the virus in the infected cells. As there is no loss of this lymphokine in urine, the levels of it continue to increase in the body with continuation of the autoimmune urine therapy. Thus the longer one fasts with autoimmune urine therapy, the better the chances are of eliminating AIDS. Autoimmune urine therapy and hyperthermia also enhances the T8 cell activity. This leads to destruction of HIV-infected cells.

25. Enhances the activity of the complement system: Autoimmune urine therapy and hyperthermia plays an important role in enhancing the activity of the complement system. Complements are protein enzymes. They are integral parts of the immune system and circulate in the blood, lymph, and tissues in an inactive form. The complements are responsible for enhancing and amplifying the affects of the immune defense system. Urate crystals are known to stimulate complements.

Likewise, autoimmune urine therapy (AUT), along with fasting and hyperthermia activates the complement system and increases their production from liver and other cells. It will help to activate the antibodies and antigen-antibody complexes, which in turn will bind with complements in blood. This reaction will set in motion a cascade of reactions resulting in enzyme formation. This will result in the formation of multiple antiparasitic, antibacterial, and antiviral products against AIDS, HIV-infected cells, opportunistic infections and cancers. They help to neutralize the circulating HIV. Complements coat the HIV-infected cells to be destroyed by phagocytic cells and T8 killer cells. In the same fashion opportunistic infections and Kaposi sarcomas are also eliminated.

26. Produces the antibodies against AIDS cofactors which enhance the disease: Dr. Shyh-Ching Lo M.D., and his associates (Armed Forces Institute of Pathology) have demonstrated a cofactor associated with HIV infection. It is called "virus like infectious agent" (VLIA). This is supposed to act as a catalyst in the development of AIDS. Syphilis, HHV-6 virus and many other factors associated with AIDS have been blamed for the development of the disease. The HIV virus without VLIA is said to be harmless (JAMA, 1989, vol. 261, p. 3361). If such cofactors are found, the vaccines and drugs that are being tested for AIDS based purely on HIV as the causative agent will be ineffective. That is why autoimmune urine therapy and hyperthermia is much more effective than any other form of therapy or vaccines. Practicing autoimmune urine therapy will result in the production of antibodies against VLIA and against other unidentified co-factors which turns HIV into an AIDS-causing virus. Hyperthermia neutralizes and/or eliminates the effect of co-factors. It enhances the output of co-factors. When fed back results in production of antibodies against co-factors.

27. Increases antibodies against HIV (Fig. 5, 6, 7): During total autoimmune urine therapy and hyperthermia with fasting, large amounts of antigenic material (HIV) and antibodies and their broken-down products are fed back. There is hardly any loss of antigens or antibodies from the body. This results in intense stimulation of immune defense system to produce antibodies. The broken down antibodies in urine provide the raw material to build more antibodies with ease. These two factors lead to increased levels of antibodies against the HIV. This results in eradication of the viruses and virus-infected cells.

28. Autoimmune urine therapy is like old broth in which the virus cannot Thrive: Total autoimmune urine therapy with fasting, hyperthermia, is a must to achieve the goal of eradicating AIDS infection. This method acts like Pasteur's old broth. Microbes do not survive in old broth. The whole human body is like a broth or culture media. Hyperthermia, fasting and AUT makes the human body like a old broth in which the microbes cannot thrive. The viruses and HIV-infected cells die like the microbes in old culture media observed by Louis Pasteur almost 100 years ago. They in turn stimulate the immune system.

29. Enhances the transfer factors which rebuilds immune system: Dr. John T. Carey (JAMA 1987, vol. 258, p. 3515) has shown improvements in immune system after injection of the Transfer Factor (TF). TF was pooled from HIV positive lymphadenopathy volunteer's blood. Improvements in the immune system were shown by acquisition of skin test responses, increased production of lymphocytes and increased natural killer cell activity. Immunity to HIV is probably transferred through leukocyte dialysate. The urine of AIDS patients also contains transfer factor. Hyperthermia enhances the output of TF. Thus, AUT with its transfer factors helps in rebuilding the devastated immune system in AIDS patients, as described by Dr. Carey. Urine is far superior to the transfer factor obtained from pooled blood. It is more specific and does not have any adverse affects on the body.

30. Neutralizes TAT gene by antibodies against it and inhibits AIDS virus growth: The AIDS virus carries a tat gene. When this gene is activated in an infected cell, the protein it encodes enters the cell nucleus and a segment of the viral genome called the promotor. This results in massive reproduction of the HIV virus. This massive replication kills the infected cell (T4 cells mostly). The tat protein can enter mammalian cells in culture. We do not know whether the same thing happens inside the AIDS patient's body. If it does, it is an active stimulator of HIV production inside the cells. There are signs that the tat cell protein may be descended from a normal cellular gene (Scientific America, March, 1989).

The blood of AIDS patient frequently contains antibodies to tat protein. During AUT and hyperthermia tat antigen is fed back through the gut and picked up by the immune cells, resulting in the production of tat antibodies. These antibodies neutralize tat genes. This dramatically reduces the viral replication inside the cell. This results in reduction in infection of newly-formed cells. The immune system cells gain an upper hand, resulting in control or elimination of HIV infection and AIDS.

31. Slows down viral growth by VPU gene expression: A ninth HIV gene named viral protein (VPU) has been discovered (Nature, 1988, vol. 333, p. 504). Why this virus has so many genes and what role they play in infected cells may take time to answer. The VPU gene is said to play a role in slowing down the virus. Hyperthermia, antiviral drugs and AUT encourages the expression of this gene and thus slows down the virus's growth and activity. By practicing total autoimmune urine therapy (TAUT) with fasting, any VPU that is being lost in the urine is fed back to the body. This in turn increases the body levels of VPU. These genes act on the virus and reduce their activity and effectiveness.

32. Slows the AIDS virus core antibody which keeps AIDS suppressed (Fig. 11): There are two types of antibodies produced in response to HIV infection: (1) Antibodies against the HIV envelope, (2) Antibodies against the core of the virus. The antibody usually develop to P24, P17, envelope gp 41, precursor of gag proteins, and reverse transcriptase. As the disease progresses antibodies to the HIV core antigen decline and even disappear. This is associated with an increase in levels of core antigens such as P24. Thus, P24 antigen test may be an important predictor of the clinical course of the disease. Lowering P24 antibodies takes place during asymptomatic or latent period of infection. Low P24 antigens also indicate the effectiveness of the AZT therapy. They decrease or disappear as the clinical disease develops and are associated with an elevation of P24 antigen (Human retrovirus and diseases they cause 1988, excerpta medica, Elsvier Publishing Co.). The patients who are asymptomatic have high levels of antibodies to the core and envelope. In patients with symptoms only antibodies to core antigens decrease or disappear. Lack of antibody to core antigen, low levels of CD4 and T4 lymphocytes are all predictors of poor outcome.

During hyperthermia, drugs therapy and autoimmune urine therapy, core antibodies and antibodies against reverse transcriptase will not go down due to constant intake of urine. They increase as autoimmune urine therapy continues. The level of CD4 receptors also increases. This would provide a locus for attachment of the AIDS virus. This results in a small number of HIV virus attacking lymphocytes. The HIV envelope antibodies also increase due to feeding back of urine. AUT attacks this deadly virus on all fronts to eliminates the disease.

33. Hyperthermia, antiviral drugs and AUT disrupts the action of polymerase, ribonuclease and Integrase, thus preventing HIV from changing into DNA: The viral reverse transcriptase consists of enzyme DNA polymerase and ribonuclease. DNA polymerase makes the first strand of the DNA, a copy of viral RNA. Then the ribonuclease destroys the viral the RNA. Then the polymerase makes a second copy of DNA. Now the viral genetic information is in the form of double- stranded DNA. A third enzyme called integrase splices the HIV genome and integrates it into host DNA. This integrated viral DNA is called a provirus. Every time the cell divides, this viral DNA also divides along with the cell DNA.

Hyperthermia, antiviral drugs and AUT helps to disrupt the activity of the above three enzyme and prevents the production of viral DNA and its integration into host cell DNA.

The end of the viral genome (long terminal repeats) directs the enzymes belonging to the host cell to copy DNA of the integrated virus into RNA. One type of RNA provides viral RNA. Another type, called messenger RNA, guides the host cell machinery to produce structural proteins and enzymes of the new virus. These two types of RNA migrate to the inside of the cell membrane. It attaches to it with the help of a fatty acid. An enzyme, a protease, cuts the protein chain and cleaves other enzymes (polymerase, ribonuclease and integrate) from long precursor molecules. Hyperthermia antiviral drugs with autoimmune urine therapy inhibits the fatty acid and protease activity. This results in a collection of large amounts of viral precursor material inside the cell without a virus. It is like an automobile engine disassembled. It won't work. When patient undergoes hyperthermia, these virus packets of cells are destroyed and viruses denatured.

34. Increased interferon alfa which inhibits the release of reverse transcriptase: Studies by Drs. Anthony Fauci and Guido Poli (JAMA 1989, vol. 262, p. 17) found that interferon alfa inhibits the release of reverse transcriptase and viral antigen into culture media of HIV-1 infected lymphocytes. It also suppressed the production and release of whole HIV virions, and reduced the number of infectious viral particles. Thus, by combining AZT with interferon alfa, they prevented replication of HIV in newly-infected cells and their release. Hyperthermia, autoimmune urine therapy with its contents of interferon alfa (combined with small doses of AZT) will act similarly. I recommend combining AUT with small doses of AZT or any other antiviral, antibacterial, or anti cancer drugs and hyperthermia as an effective therapy. AZT is excreted in urine (14% intact, 75% as metabolized GAZT). This is taken back in AUT. That is why the dose of AZT has to be reduced. Refeeding of AZT and its metabolized products, and interferon alfa during AUT will prevent replication of the HIV virus and its release from the infected cells. It is an effective method for achieving a complete cure with the least amount of AZT toxicity. Other drugs can also be used in small doses along with AUT to combat opportunistic infection and cancers associated with AIDS.

Recently (July 1990), there are reports from Kenya indicating that ingesting small amounts of interferon will cure/or curtail AIDS. These studies are interesting because, I strongly believe that the urine of AIDS patient contain interferons, specially so the urine of patients undergoing hyperthermia therapy. When AUT is practiced, these interferons will help the body fight AIDS virus and eliminate the infection. Due to heat during hyperthermia, the production of lymphokines, interferons, antibodies,etc will increase many folds. Thus hyperthermia is a good adjunct therapy for AIDS and other incurable,chronic diseases. I believe that hyperthermia along with AUT will cure rabies -a deadly disease as well as many viral, bacterial and chronic diseases.

35. Acts as nonspecific immune system booster: Immune boosting typhoid vaccine can be taken under supervision of a physician once a week for 3-4 months. It helps in boosting the immune system the same way as the BCG vaccination used in the treatment of some kinds of cancer. Urine coming out after hyperthermia is a far better nonspecific immune system stimulator than the typhoid vaccine.

36. Produces changes in AIDS viral genetic material (Fig. 11): The AIDS virus and host cells produce many types of proteins during hyperthermia and AUT with fasting. There is no supply of protein from the outside. The cells have to scramble from within to get an adequate supply. In the scramble, the body cells and the HIV start behaving erratically and produce proteins with structures a bit different from their original proteins especially after hyperthermia. Many types of antibodies are produced during total autoimmune urine therapy (TAUT). Antibodies are proteins. They become easy food proteins. So in the game of survival, the viruses and the virus infested cells start using the antibodies and the antigens for their protein needs. The virus gets confused and starts using these proteins. This will result in changes in the structure of the replicated viral RNA and DNA. These viruses produced by the altered proteins will not reproduce. Even if they reproduce, the progeny are harmless. They loose their ability to destroy the immune system T4 cells. Even if they reproduce, they will not be harmful to the body. This ultimately leads to elimination of the AIDS virus in the body and a cure for the AIDS sufferers. Hyperthermia augments this process.

37. Training of Lymphocytes to Attack AIDS Virus, opportunistic infections and Cancers: In a recent study, Dr. N.Osband of Boston University School of Medicine removed the lymphocytes from the body and trained them to recognize and attack caner cells and return them to the body. These lymphocytes are called autolymphocytes (ATL). This kind of therapy has prolonged the life of kidney cancer patients 2.5 times longer. The kidney cancer affects about 25000 people and kills 10,000 people every year in US (Lancet, April 1990).

During autoimmune urine therapy with hyperthermia, the antigens and various lymphokines output is enhanced. They are absorbed from the intestines. These substances come in contact with the lymphocytes in the wall of the intestines. By continuously fasting and feeding urine these substances come in close contact with the lymphocytes. They get stimulated to multiply and trained to recognize the viruses, protozoa, fungus, cancer cells etc and kill them. The human body is the best culture media there is. It will help to develop these autolymphocytes which will fight the diseases. Total autoimmune urine therapy with fasting produces autolymphocytes the same way as produced by Dr. Osband experiments to fight the cancer or even better.

38. Heating the body (hyperthermia-read chapter 1) in conjunction with AUT melts the cell membrane of the infected cells and denatures virus, inhibits the reverse transcriptase and other enzymes needed for viral reproduction, increases the antigen output in the urine which will in turn increase antibody output (Fig. 1, 2): We have known for decades that the cancer does disappear after an infection or and elevation of body temperature. There are reports of treating the cancer by artificially elevating the body temperature. This results in the destruction of the cancer cells which are heat sensitive. We tried this method in our hospital on advanced cancers. We know that the HIV is heat sensitive. So is also the enzyme reverse transcriptase. This enzyme is responsible for viral multiplication. Raising the body temperature will kill many of these viruses and destroy, reduce or alter the enzyme needed for it's survival. The host cells that are infected with HIV virus also die. It will kill many HIV reservoir cells. The cell membranes in these cancer cells are weakened by the AIDS virus. With elevated body temperature, these cells simply rupture and release the viruses in to circulation. Thus, the body stores of the virus are destroyed. The enemy, the HIV virus, is exposed to the body immune system. The heat that permeates the entire body will kill all the weak cells that are infected with the virus. These viruses are excreted from urine in the billions. They are again fed back to the system, which in turn stimulate the immune system as described before (read chapter 9). Thus, combining the heat therapy with autoimmune urine therapy along antiviral agents can assure a possible cure.

It is interesting to note that the patients under hyperthermia therapy put out many ounces of urine containing all the disease-causing viruses, dead cells, important body proteins from the disintegrated cells, electrolytes, hormones, minerals, etc., in proper proportions. When these material are fed back in physiological proportions, it will not affect the body adversely. It is better to feed the urine back, which is close to our body fluids, than to give large amounts of intravenous fluids to replace it during hyperthermia.

Large amounts of urine is produced after hyperthermia. This primarily due to increased blood circulation (elevated cardiac output). It does not contain the toxic metabolic substances. It is rich in antigenic material, lymphokines, basic building materia, electrolytes, metal, etc. What a elixir of life, if we give it back to our body which was produced by hard working 75 trillion cells in our body. Due to increased force of circulation and heat, many of the microbes, antigens and antibodies are freed, circulated and come out in the urine also. Hyperthermia is like a draino for cleaning the clogged sewers.

After the hyperthermia, there is likelihood of HIV test becoming negative. This can happen because, the immunoglobulin and the circulating antigens are destroyed by the heat. The heat increases the urine output. This can result in washing of the antibodies out in the urine, resulting in reduction of their titer. It is important to note that the AIDS virus is incorporated in the genetic material of the cell and could not be destroyed unless the cell infected with the virus is also destroyed. Hyperthermia alone can give temporary cure, but the disease is more likely to relapse after certain time unless it is combined with the autoimmune urine therapy and possible other antiviral agents.

Another interesting aspect of hyperthermia is that the co-factors which are said play an important role are destroyed by elevated temperature. Thus the virus will stay within the cell dormant for long periods due to lack of cofacotrs. Once it gets the cofacotrs, the virus gets triggered and begin to multiply. AUT, hyperthermia and antiviral HIV drugs can eliminate cells containing viruses which act as reservoir as well free floating viruses. To eliminate AIDS, the cells acting as HIV reservoirs has to be eliminated.

I believe that many electrolyte imbalances we produce and treat them with parenteral administration of artificially made fluids can be cut totally if the patients are fed with their own urine during surgery and after surgery, in the intensive care units. This therapy will save the patients life and maintain the body in proper balance at no cost. This therapy is a must in patients' who have head injuries and are unconscious.

If I get opportunity I would like the body temperature of the of HIV positive patients and AIDS patients (and patients with viral, bacterial, fungal, spirochetal, or any other unknown infections and acute or chronic incurable diseases) to be raised to 40-41.8° C. by using radiant heat method or induce mild to moderate hyperthermia by using dry sauna, hot tubs, and jacuzzi, (not by extracorporeal heating) for 1-2-4 hours. Hyperthermia may have to be repeated about half dozen time. Hyperthermia by itself may not the cure the disease. It is a great adjunct therapy. Feed the entire urine back during hyperthermia. This method has a good possibility of cure. When this mode of treatment is followed in the HIV positive patient's, they may never develop the full-blown AIDS. All I am going to say again is, give me an opportunity; with autoimmune urine therapy combined with antiviral drugs (in small doses) and hyperthermia therapy, total remission of the disease or cure is possible.

There is a possibility of curing rabies, leprosy, tuberculosis, leukemia, Alzheimer's, multiple sclerosis, cancers, asthma, autoimmune diseases, heart and blood vessels diseases, psoriasis lupus, skin diseases, leprosy, kidney diseases, obesity (cellulite), drugs and alcohol abdication, and many other incurable diseases with this method of therapy (heating the body and combining it with autoimmune urine therapy, and small amounts of disease specific drugs if needed).

39. Flushing or Neutralizing Neurotoxic Metabolites of Tryptophan Contribution to Dementia: The latest report indicates that the AIDS dementia may be linked to a metabolite of Tryptophan (JAMA 264:305-306.1990). Quinolinic acid is a neurotoxic convulsant metabolite of tryptophan activated by interferon gamma. It raises as much as 1000 folds in AIDS patients with dementia. It is also elevated after common cold virus to lenti virus infections. It is likely most of the viral infections including rabies, it is increased contributing to mental symptoms. "Cant think properly" during cold can be attributed to this metabolite associated mental changes. It binds to nerve receptors (N-methyl-D-aspartate receptors) which are involved in normal neurotransmission, neural regulation, memory, and synaptic plasticity.

Quinolinic acid can also induce seizures and nerve cell death. The levels of these metabolites go up with AIDS dementia and opportunistic infections of the central nervous system such as toxoplasmosis, progressive multifocal leukoencephalopathy, lymphomas,etc.

Theenzyme(indoleamine-2,-3-dioxygenase,IDL)whichconverts tryptophan to quinolinic acid increases in the lungs and brain. So the metabolism shifts from the liver to brain. Hyperthermia breaks the blood brain barrier and flushes out all the quinolinic acid and neutralizes the IDL enzyme which converts tryptophan into this toxic substance. By reducing the enzyme IDL and Quinolinic acid content of the brain, hyperthermia and AUT will reduce or eliminate AIDS or other infection associated dementia including AIDS and rabies.

It is quite likely, that after general anesthesia, Quinolinic acid level goes up due to inhibition of indoleamine-2,-3-dioxygenase by most general anesthetics. This can have effect on memory we often see after general anesthesia. We often see that the AIDS patient need less anesthetics and their wake up and recall time is somewhat prolonged can also attributed to raise in Quinolinic acid.

Read Chapters 1, 7, 8, 9, 10, 14, 15, 16, 17, 19 and 20 to understand how hyperthermia and autoimmune urine therapy (AUT) works in the body. Almost all the explanations given in these chapters, also apply here wherever pertinent.

Autoimmune Urine Therapy and Hyperthermia Outlines in People Who Are HIV Positive (as well as other microbial and acute and chronic diseases) with No Sign and Symptoms of AIDS or ARC (Fig. 8)

1. Practice total autoimmune urine therapy during and after hyperthermia for one to two weeks with complete fasting.
2. Then start eating high energy, low calorie, vitamin rich food.
3. Drink morning urine completely every day along with a full glass of water. Use water without fluoride. Fluoride has shown to prevent repair of damaged DNA within the cells. Drink an additional glass of urine, one at mid-noon and another in the evening.
4. Collect the rest of the urine in a bowl and apply all over the body including the scalp for 1-3 hours a day.
5. Take a dropper and apply fresh urine drops into your nose, eyes and ears.
6. Gargle your mouth with urine 4-6 times a day. Keep the urine in the mouth 5 to 10 minutes at a time. This will prevent all the afflictions of the mouth, including hairy leukoplakia, oral thrush, stomatitis, etc. Brush your teeth with urine after meals.
7. Take vitamins as indicated below.
8. Eat vegetables, especially carrots, spinach, squash, beans, peas, lettuce, peppers. Eat fruits (different kinds) once every day. Add garlic and onion to your vegetables. Include condiments and herbs.
9. Use one teaspoonful of bran 1-2 times a day.

10. Do not eat diary products and food rich in animal fats, such as hamburgers. Eat fish and fowl. Eat lean red meat once a week. Replace your meat with soybean products (tofu) twice a week.
11. Avoid fried foods.
12. Avoid palm and coconut oil completely.
13. Eat cold-pressed, unrefined, fresh linseed oil mixed with cottage cheese (1 to 2 tablespoonsful a day).
14. Exercise moderately. Walking for 45 minutes, 3 to 5 days a week.
15. Do not smoke, drink alcohol, or take any drugs.
16. Practice safe sex. Let your partner know you are HIV positive. Continue with your social life and profession.
17. Rest well. Take a 15-20 minute nap after meals and get a good night's sleep.
18. Attend spiritual gatherings. It can give you strength. There are studies that show that a positive attitude can enhance the immune system.
19. If you develop any infections, get them treated. Do not linger.
20. Get tested for syphilis. If tests are positive, get treatment. Claims have been made that the syphilis organism, not the HIV virus may be the primary agent in AIDS. I do not believe in this concept. However, it may play a role in triggering the reproduction of AIDS virus (cofactor). Many ARC patients treated solely for syphilis have showed improvement. The test should be done using the FTA-ABS test or the MHA-TP test, instead of commonly used VDRL test (AIDS and Syphilis, North Atlantic Books). The existence of syphilis can aggravate the AIDS condition.
21. Small dose of AZT or any other antiviral drug in the horizon can be combined with this therapy.
22. Heating the body (Hyperthermia as discussed before using dry sauna and hot tubs), along with AUT and AZT should be seriously considered. Hyperthermia may have to be repeated many times.

If you continue the above guidelines, you will be free from developing AIDS or ARC or any other disease associated with it.

You will have a worry-free life. This therapy can be used for all HIV positive groups, including hemophiliacs, pregnant women, children, and adults, without any exception.

Autoimmune Urine Therapy and Hyperthermia for Those Who Have ARC and AIDS

1. Follow the regimen as described above
2. Total autoimmune urine therapy (TAUT) along with fasting, antiviral agents and hyperthermia, should be practiced for 3-6 weeks at a time.
3. This is followed by 2-3 weeks of above described food and vitamin regimen along with prophylactic autoimmune urine therapy (PAUT).
4. Again, follow two weeks of total autoimmune urine therapy. Followed by three weeks of prophylactic autoimmune urine therapy.
5. Then practice one week TAUT followed by four weeks of PAUT.
6. Continue PAUT all your life. Practice one week of TAUT for eight weeks of PAUT.
7. During TAUT, supplemental vitamins may have to be taken if there is deficiency.
8. The period of TAUT can be altered according to the condition of the patient.
9. Combine TAUT with hyperthermia and other antiviral drugs.

Combining AZT, ddI with AUT and Hyperthermia for HIV positive, ARC and AIDS

This can be of value if it is done under a physician's supervision. Urine after AZT and ddI therapy looks like muddy water and has the smell of drugs. The patient already has nausea and vomiting due to the drug. Drinking the urine may be difficult. In such cases, insert a soft, small size (10-12 french size) feeding tube. Pour the urine into a clean fluid bottle and attach the drip at the end of the feeding tube. Medical pumps can also be used to feed the urine. These nasogastric tubes can be tolerated for months without any discomfort. Autoimmune urine therapy with fasting results in trituration, dilution with agitation which will enhance the effectiveness of AZT and other drugs.

It is important to remember that urine contains 14% of AZT unchanged and 75% metabolized AZT as GAZT. Refeeding the AZT for months can have severe adverse reactions. When you start autoimmune urine therapy, start with approximately 250 mg every 4 hours for two to three days. Then do not take it for two to three days. Then again, restart the therapy. Because of refeeding the AZT and its metabolic products, you may have to doctor the dose according to the reaction. If you develop a severe reaction, stop AZT, drink urine along with water till you feel comfortable, and again restart.

I have not treated any AIDS patient as a primary care physician. I have taken care of them on the operating room table during anesthesia. So I cannot tell how I would tailor the dose. I will go on the basis of the day-to-day condition of the patient. Because of TAUT, the dose of AZT need to be reduced. All you need per day may be 25 to 50 mg every six hours. This is something you have to work out. Do not stop autoimmune urine therapy because the urine looks or smells different after tking drugs. This practice will be continued for 4-6 weeks followed by PAUT, with a reduced dose of AZT or no AZT. Usually 75% of the AZT is absorbed from the intestines. During TAUT, due to lack of any food material coating the intestines most of the AZT is absorbed. This is also one reason for reducing the dose.

It has been known that anticancer drugs are more effective after subjecting them by to hyperthermia.(Cancer 38, 279-287, 1976). Same way antimicrobial drugs more effective even in smaller concentrations after hyperthermia.

External massage should continue everyday for one to two hours. Follow the same regimen as described for HIV patients. There are patients who cannot tolerate nasogastric tubes, because their esophagus is affected by the disease. In such cases, let a surgeon perform a gastrostomy and feed the urine, water and nutrition through that tube (see Fig. 8). Autoimmune urine therapy ends the problem of anemia caused by AZT, because urine contains hormones which stimulate the red bone marrow to produce more red blood cells, as well as white blood cells of the immune system.

Autoimmune Urine Therapy, Hyperthermia and drugs for HIV Positive Newborns and Children

These children need to grow and develop. It is difficult to collect urine until the child is 3-5 years old. The only way to start autoimmune urine therapy in these children is by inserting a catheter (Foley) into the bladder. Collect the urine at elected intervals. Feed it through a nasogastric feeding tube (see Fig. 8). Start with 3-7 days of total autoimmune urine therapy (TAUT) followed by prophylactic autoimmune urine therapy for 3-7 days (PAUT). Combine AUT with hyperthermia.

For children, time under hyperthermia may have to be cut down compared to adults. Continue alternating TAUT and PAUT. Feeding morning urine is a must. The whole procedure is simple. The child will grow better than a normal child. It will nourish and flourish. Once the child can pass the urine, you can train the child to pass urine into a clean bowl. Then feed it through the nasogastric tube or make the child drink the urine. Autoimmune urine therapy should continue the rest of child's life or until the disease is completely eradicated. Always feed the baby with plenty of water with urine.

Autoimmune Urine Therapy, Hyperthermia and drugs for Opportunistic Infections and Cancers

HIV infection itself does not kill AIDS patient. It is the opportunistic infections, which are attacking the defenseless body that claim your life. It is like a termite attacking a dead tree. It is very important to remember that autoimmune urine therapy with hyperthermia and antimicrobial drugs are very effective against bacterial, protozoal, fungal, viral, spirocheta infections and various types of cancers. These opportunistic infections do not start with full force. First, there are a small number of organisms which get a foothold in the body. Then, they begin to multiply and spread.

If the immune defense system is strong, the invading organisms are eliminated by it. As there is total breakdown of the immune system in AIDS patients, they begin to grow and spread uncontrolled. As the number of microbes attacking the vital organs increases, their normal functioning are affected. As the infection becomes overwhelming, the affected organs fail, resulting in death.

Begin autoimmune urine therapy with hyperthermia when there is no opportunistic infection, when AIDS virus is gradually destroying the immune system. The microorganisms are getting a foothold in the body. These organisms are still attacked by the existing immune system and many of these microbes are killed. Hyperthermia kills billions of these opportunistic microbes and flushed through the urine. Their antigenic material comes out in the urine as well as circulates in the body. Such antigenic material containing urine is taken orally. This antigen is picked up by the immune defense cells. Antibodies are produced against the microbes. In the same fashion, as the cancers begin to develop, the destroyed cancer cells and their causative agents are excreted in urine. When such urine is taken orally, it results in the development of immunity. It will eliminate further development as well the existing cancer.

A time may come when we subject a person who are predisposed to cancer, heart disease and other incurrable disease to hyperthermia and AUT as a prophylactic measure.

With pneumocystis carinii pneumonia (PCP), the antibodies are produced against this protozoa. These antibodies attack it and coat it with circulating antibodies. Many of these protozoa die in the attack and during hyperthermia. Those which are coated with the antibodies become more palatable to the attacking white blood cells. They are devoured and digested by super charged white blood cells. The macrophages swallow these parasites, partially digest them, and present them to lymphocytes (as antigen). The lymphocytes start producing T and B cells. The B cells differentiate into plasma cells and specific B clone cells. The plasma cells produce large amount of antibodies.

The stimulated T cells differentiate into T4 and T8 cells. T4 cells produce interlukin-II and alpha-interferon which increase the entire immune cells activity. T8 cells directly attack parasites and parasite containing cells (as well as cancer cells, leprosy infected cells and HIV-infected cells) and kill them. AUT acts on other opportunistic infections of AIDS in a similar fashion. The same phenomenon takes place in early cancers treated with AUT and hyperthermia. Before these infections and tumors find a foothold and damage the body, they are eliminated by practicing autoimmune urine therapy and hyperthermia. That is why, by continuously practicing total and prophylactic autoimmune urine therapy, the chances for developing opportunistic infections and cancers is eliminated.

If hyperthermia is not available, enter into dry sauna or hot water tub for more than 30 minutes with high temperature setting one to three times a week can have very beneficial effects. It can help to eliminate opportunistic infections and kaposi sarcoma same way as hyperthermia. AUT should be continued even during mild to moderate hyperthermia.

If a patient is undergoing treatment, autoimmune urine therapy hyperthermia can only help. The person taking any antibacterial, antifungal, antiprotozoal, and anticancer therapy agent should continue. However, the dose of these drugs must to be reduced. Proper monitoring for development of any toxic symptoms should be kept in mind. Many of these drugs are excreted in urine unchanged or as metabolized degradation products. Drinking urine will feed back some of these drugs excreted in urine. That is why it is important to reduce the dose of these drugs. Some of these drugs are highly toxic and expensive. During autoimmune urine therapy, the dose of these drugs being reduced results in a reduction of cost, as well as reduction or elimination of toxic effects.

In conclusion, practicing autoimmune urine therapy from the very beginning (as soon as you are tested HIV positive) along with hyperthermia and antimicrobial drugs will prevent the development of severe opportunistic infections and various kinds of tumors. Thus, AUT will prolong the life of HIV positive and AIDS patients. Even if the infection and cancers do develop, they will not be as severe. They will be mild type which the body defenses can handle with the help of drugs and urine therapy. I would like to combine AUT, hyperthermia along with antimicrobial agents in treating the opportunistic infections.

Autoimmune Urine Therapy and Hyperthermia for AIDS or other Disease Associated Lesions of the Mouth, Lips, and Digestive Tract

The best therapy for any and all oral and nasal lesions (on the tongue, lips, cheek, palate, nose, and pharynx) is application of hot compressors soaked in urine, AUT and hyperthermia. Save some of the morning urine in a clean container. Gargle the mouth every 2-4 hours with morning urine if there is a lesion in the mouth. Warm the urine and gargle, (do not boil) as the day passes. For lesions on the lip, apply urine repeatedly soaked in a cotton swab or gauge, or small sponge. Hairy leukoplakia and thrush will disappear with this therapy. The coating of these lesion may have to be scraped using a hard toothbrush or plastic tongue scraper before applying urine packs. You will be amazed how effective urine is for these lesions.

Besides the above-mentioned methods showing how the urine cures or curtail AIDS and other diseases, urine contains urea, nonprotein nitrogen and creatinine which are antiviral in nature. They do not allow viruses to multiply. Every time urine is consumed, levels of these components are elevated in the blood due to absorption from the gut. This inhibits the viral activity and prevent the newly released viral particles from attacking the healthy T4 lymphocytes (AIDS virus main target). Further as the urine passes through the esophagus and the gut, various antiviral constituents of urine coat the inner lining of the mucous membrane. As these constituents are absorbed from inside the gut, all the layers of the entire digestive system are coated with the urine. Thus, there is increased levels of urea, NPN, creatinine, etc., in these areas. They in turn prevent any bacterial, fungal, viral, and protozoal infections of the digestive system. They also reduce the chance of gut cells changing into cancer cells. Thus the insides of the body which comes in contact with urine get cleaned the same way as the lesions of the mouth and skin are healed by external urine application.

AUT and hyperthermia for Kaposi's Sarcoma and Skin Afflictions in AIDS (Fig. 5, 9, 10)

There is a possibility that the Kaposi's sarcoma is a form of immune response. It is nature's way of protecting the body. That is probably one of the reasons why AIDS patients with Kaposi sarcoma live longer than other patients. Follow the autoimmune urine therapy with hyperthermia as described for AIDS in chapter 1 in this chapter. Initially entering into dry sauna or hot tub with high temperature setting for more than 30 minutes can completely prevent development of Kaposi sarcoma. Apply urine on the lesions many hours and repeatedly especially after coming out of sauna. If one has a large lesion, apply hot urine soaked gauze on it and keep it wet with urine for hours. Continue the therapy for many months. You will ultimately get the benefit. For all skin lesions of AIDS, external application and hyperthermia should be practiced. Applying warmed 1-2 day old urine for all types of skin afflictions is more helpful.

It may be important to enter a dry sauna chamber with the highest temperature setting for more than 30 minutes immediately after applying urine. The elevated skin temperature along with urine can kill many microbes, precancerous and cancerous cells. There are known cases of cancer cures when body temperature have been elevated artificially or due to secondary infections. Combined autoimmune urine therapy, external applications of urine and raising the skin temperature to the maximum in a dry sauna, hot tubs or by hyperthermia can cure all skin afflictions, including Kaposi's sarcoma. Urine application, dry sauna and hyperthermia helps to stimulate the activity of Langerhans cells and keratinocytes of the skin. They enhance the immune system and eliminates skin lesions. Read Chapter 1,8,9,10,18,19 for more details.

Foods During Hyperthermia and Autoimmune Urine Therapy

There are literally hundreds of books describing how to eat, what to eat to cure every known disease and live a long healthy life. As autoimmune urine therapy is a new subject, we want to make it sure that the person follows certain guidelines. Urine is "The water with life". It contains many nutrients, salts, vitamins, and hormones needed by the body (see Chapter 7). Do not overload the system by taking large quantities of vitamins, minerals, and food during autoimmune urine therapy. Observe moderation in all phases of your life including the food you eat, the water you drink, and the work you do.

1. **Foods You Should Eat:** Whole grains, (oat, bran, millet, buckwheat, brown rice, etc.), skimmed milk, fruits of all kinds, fiber-rich vegetables (raw, steamed or cooked), freshly prepared carrot juice, sprouted alfalfa and moong beans, fish (salmon, mackerel, sardine) and poultry (three times a week), defatted cottage cheese, tofu (soybean product), natural spring water, brown sugar, all kinds of nuts (eat two to three whole, overnight-soaked almonds every day) yogurt, lentils, beans, peas.

2. **Foods to Avoid Completely:** Sausage, pork, processed meat, bacon, white sugar, pastries, puddings, donuts, shell fish, processed food such as chips, apple juice (has too much sugar), cheese, fried foods, refined flour, coconut and palm oil, dairy butter or lard, fluorides, foods containing artificial chemicals, sweeteners, food additives including mono sodium glutamate (MSG), lead, monostearates, tryptophan concentrates, etc.

3. **Drinking, Smoking, Inhaling:** Carbonated drinks, coffee, alcohol, smoking tobacco or marijuana, crack, or any other addictive drugs, distilled water, water with fluorides, artificial sweeteners, including Nutrasweet (aspertane), etc., should be avoided.

4. **Vitamins That Boost Immune Systems and Health:** Vitamin A, in the form of carrot juice, Vitamin B complex tablets three times a day, Vitamin C 500mg three times a day, Vitamin D, 400IU a day, Vitamin E, 500mg two times a day, slow release Niacin (B6) 500mg two times a day, Vitamin B12, 100 mcg a day, Folate, 400 mcg a day, Omega 3 Fish Oil 1 capsule twice a day, Choline and Methionine, Aspartate, Vitamin P etc should be included in daily regimes of diet.

5. **Trace Metals:** Zinc, selenium, magnesium, molybdenum (found in cauliflower), etc., should be included in the diet. Many AIDS patients have zinc deficiency. It is an important metal needed in production of hormones, enzyme activities and healing.

6. **Spices in Your Foods:** Garlic, onion, cardamon (1/16 th seed), clove (1/2 to 1 clove), ginger, green and red pepper, black pepper, coriander, cumin seeds, mustard seeds, cinnamon, asfotida, tamarind, turmeric, etc., should all be included in the diet in moderate amounts.

Immune System Boosters for HIV Positive and AIDS

Most of the above-described vitamins and foods boost the immune system. In addition, include fruits like pineapple (rich in bromelin, which stimulates muscles and glands), spirulin, coenzyme Q, zinc, magnesium, molybdenum, (abundant in cauliflower) selenium, bee pollen, honey (a tablespoonful a day), linseed oil, ginseng,etc.

I will start the day with one teaspoonful of cold pressed, fresh, unrefined linseed oil mixed with 1/2 cup defatted cottage cheese (cottage cheese can be replaced by oatmeal). Or you could drink a glass of skimmed milk mixed with one teaspoonful of linseed oil. This is followed an hour later by a fruit (different fruits every day). For lunch, have steamed vegetables and brown rice with mixed spices. Have an afternoon herbal tea or buttermilk or freshly prepared carrot juice. For supper eat two to six ounces of fish, chicken or turkey along with a salad, and steamed vegetables. You can add flaxseed (linseed) to your food preparation.

I am not going to give you a menu on how to prepare these foods. Select the food ingredients from the above list. Choose according to your own needs. Prepare the meals to your taste. Take all the vitamins, essential minerals, and immune system boosters every day along with your food.

As you are practicing autoimmune urine therapy, the body gets plenty of electrolytes from urine (sodium, potassium, chloride calcium phosphates and magnesium, etc). If your urine tastes salty, reduce your salt intake. As a rule, restrict salt intake. If you have to eat red meat, choose lean, fat free cuts, about six ounces a serving.

When food faddists talk about a macrobiotic diet, they are talking about most of the above-mentioned foods eaten in small quantities. No meat is allowed in this diet. Macrobiotic is the art of lengthening the life span by a vegetarian diet. Vegetables are grown under natural conditions, with organic fertilizers and without chemical fertilizers. As urine itself is food, eat only small qualities of the chosen food. **AUT is the best macrobiotic diet there is. I call it Nature's Super Macrobiotic Diet with Life.**

Do I Have Proof that Autoimmune Urine Therapy, Hyperthermia and Antimicrobial Drugs Works?

I have discussed in detail how autoimmune urine therapy with or without hyperthermia and drugs can help AIDS patients. Do I have the experimental proof? The answer to that question is No. The answer to how autoimmune urine therapy and hyperthermia works is based purely on knowledge of how it cures other deadly diseases. This includes my own experiences. There are hundreds of cases of cancers, tuberculosis, skin diseases, various infectious diseases, malaria, arthritis, jaundice, leukemia, paralysis, Hodgkin's disease, gangrene, diphtheria, flu, asthma, heart diseases, arteriosclerotic vascular diseases, stroke, diabetes, colon diseases, coronary artery diseases, etc., being cured by autoimmune urine therapy. These cases were reported in two monographs. There are many reported cancers disappearing after bouts of fever. Advanced cancers have been treated with total body hyperthermia with some successes. AIDS is not cancer. So it is treatable by using hyperthermia combined with AUT and drugs.

Currently, I am preparing a book ("Hyperthermia and Autoimmune Urine Therapy-The Water with Life, Volume II") which explains scientifically why and how it works in curing various diseases. Based on my twenty-five years of research and knowledge, I do believe there is **hope in autoimmune urine therapy, drugs and hyperthermia in curing or curtailing AIDS.** AIDS patients are spending millions of dollars on cures that do not work, cures that injure the body, cures which have no scientific basis. Then why not try this therapy? It is free and easily available. You can stop therapy at any time. You do not have to consult or tell anybody about it. **Have a positive outlook; be resolute; pray to God that the autoimmune urine therapy and hyperthermia will help you; start the therapy now without delay.**

As Richard Dunne, (American Health, June 1987), director of Gay Mens Health Crisis in New York put it, "Research does not seem to understand at a feeling level the predicament of a dying person who hears of something promising. Patients ought to be offered virtually anything that holds any promise of being effective. Human beings have a right to make their own decision." I believe that autoimmune urine therapy has such a promise in AIDS and other diseases, such as cancers, leprosy, rabies, tuberculosis, multiple sclerosis, aging, Alzheimer's disease, etc.

How Long It Takes for AUT, and Hyperthermia and/or Drugs to Alleviate AIDS and the AIDS Virus?

I am not sure how long it will take to rid HIV infection and cure AIDS. I do not know of any case being treated by this method. Based on the cures of hundreds of cases of infectious diseases, cancer, asthma, cardiovascular disease, skin conditions, jaundice nephritis, etc., autoimmune urine therapy may take almost four to twelve months to cure AIDS and end HIV infection. It may have to be practiced all through life to keep HIV under control. I am of the opinion that hyperthermia enhances the effect of AUT and thus brings an early end to the disease.

Again, I am speculating on the time. The problems with viral diseases such as AIDS is that the virus gets into the genetic material of normal functioning cells of the immune defense system and other cells. Unless all the cells containing the AIDS virus are eliminated, the chances of cure of the disease are not good. On the other hand, if we keep the AIDS viral pool low, and build back the T4 lymphocyte to normal levels, the infected cells are gradually reduced and eliminated. A person can live a normal life, without being attacked and killed by opportunistic infections and cancers.

One of the interesting aspects of AIDS virus infection is that it attacks cells which are replaced by new sets of cells. None of these infected cells are permanent cells like brain or heart muscle cells. If these kinds of cells were infected, it would have been difficult to cure the disease. By attacking the cells infected, and the free floating AIDS viral particles in blood which are about to attack the new cells, we can end the disease. By combining autoimmune urine therapy, antiviral drugs, hyperthermia, proper nutrition, exercise and rest, we can achieve this goal. As we continue to fast with autoimmune urine therapy and hyperthermia, the cells infected with the AIDS virus are eliminated. The newly released viruses are attacked by the antibodies and various other mechanisms described in autoimmune urine therapy and hyperthermia. With progression of therapy, the pool or the reservoir of infected cells decreases and the healthy cells increases. Finally, we hope and pray that the entire pool of the AIDS virus and their infected cells are eliminated.

Once we start conquering the disease, we are half-way through the battle. An Englishman fasted on urine and water for 101 days to cure his blindness caused by a bee sting. The AIDS treatment may need such an approach.

You may ask how any one can fast for such long lengths of time? My answer is simple. As described before, urine contains many nutritional products which act as food. Your body energy requirements are met, if not the total calorie requirements. Even if you loose a few pounds, so what? It is important also to note that, the body does not have to spend energy to make use of these nutrients from urine. They are easily absorbed, assimilated, and used for energy needs. If a person is very sick, hyperthermia and AUT may have to be practiced under a physician's supervision. If a physician is not willing to help you start the therapy, nothing will stop you doing it on your own. Blood tests have to be performed at regular intervals. Careful watch on the vital organs functioning have to be monitored. Do whatever to stay alive. Strive hard, the cure may be closer than you think.

Give autoimmune urine therapy hyperthermia a chance.
It has many surprises in store.
Without trying, we do not know whether it works or not.
Try, Try, Try again.
Wish for a disease-free body, worry-free mind, a cost-free therapy, and a long, happy life, with grace, dignity and honor.

CHAPTER 19

AUTOIMMUNE THERAPY AND HYPERTHERMIA FOR RABIES, LEPROSY AND TUBERCULOSIS

How to Cure or Curtail Rabies, Leprosy, Tuberculosis and Other Acute and Chronic Incurable Diseases Caused by Microbes and Other Causative Agents

This book will be incomplete without describing how to treat rabies, tuberculosis and leprosy. This therapy can be adopted to other incurable diseases caused by any microbe or offending agent. Rabies like AIDS is a terminal disease. Rabies is one of the oldest disease known to mankind, compared to the AIDS of the present decade. It is referred in twenty-third century B.C., Pre-Mosaic Eshunna Code. Warm blooded animals and man are susceptible to this disease. It is transmitted to the humans mostly by dog and cat bites. Rats, squirrels, foxes, jackals, cattle and bats are also the source of this infection. The people with rabies die within two weeks after development of the symptoms. So there is not much time left to plan or find a therapy. Rabies is like a death sentence on innocent person, carried out swiftly.

Rabies is caused by a RNA virus similar to AIDS. It affects the brain and is transmitted by animal bites. It can be effectively prevented by treating the animal bite wounds and taking anti rabies vaccine. Hundreds of people die in the third world by rabies due to lack of facilities to treat animal bites and lack of proper understanding about preventive vaccines. About 20,000 people are said to die due to rabies in India alone. I worked in Communicable Disease Center of Atlanta in mid sixties on rabies and published a research paper on possible routes of transmission of rabies to the nervous system (Bull.World Hlth Org. 33: 783-794,1965,). During my study, I stuck my left index finger with a syringe full of rabies virus. I took anti rabies vaccine to prevent the development of the disease.

There are reports of two cases of rabies survival by symptomatic therapy in the literature (Ann.Intern. Med., 76:931, 1972, JAMA, 236:2751, 1976). I talked to the concerned officials in CDC to study the effect of Autoimmune Urine Therapy (AUT) in experimental animals without successes. I believe that the Autoimmune Urine Therapy combined with moderate to severe hyperthermia and intensive care of the patient has good chance of survival of most of the rabies patients. **Please give me a chance to treat these patients and prove whether my treatment works or not.**

Physicians, Please Follow these outlines on your patients if you want to save their life:

1. Admit the patient to the intensive care. Take strict measures not to come in direct contact with the patients. Adopt universal precautions. People handling the patients should take prophylactic anti rabies vaccination. If they come in contact with any body fluid from the patients complete course of antirabies vaccination is needed.
2. Paralyze the patient and insert an endotracheal tube, and breath artificially by ventilator. Start arterial line and insert a Swan Ganz catheter, Foley catheter, and a feeding tube. If some of the above monitoring facilities are not available, simple blood pressure cuff and a central venous pressure monitoring will do. Measure all the vital signs, body functions, and their response to

disease and therapy. Keep the patient paralyzed by curare and other muscle relaxants. Sedate the patient with tranquilizers, barbiturates (valium, pentothal, versed, vistaril, chloral hydrate etc).

3. Maintain proper fluid and electrolytes balance. Do not give glucose solutions unless the blood glucose is very low and has the symptoms of hypoglycemia.
4. Feed all the urine back into the digestive system through the feeding tube (see Fig. 8) with the help of a medical pump (if available) or a through a bottle or urine collecting bag attached to the feeding tube. Do not inject urine through the vein.
5. Put the patient through moderate to severe hyperthermia for 1-6 hours at a time. This may have to be done every day or every other day for 3-7 days or more. We have to tailor the time spent in hyperthermia and number of days needed according to the condition of the patient. Use the method of hyperthermia I recommend in chapter 1. Do not use extracorporeal method to induce hyperthermia. It is dangerous and life threatening. Do not over do it or under do it. This is clinical judgement call. Feed all the urine back to the patient. If the urine output is low, more fluids needs to be administered through the vein or orally. Do not over hydrate (over load with fluids) the patient. Give fluids enough to maintain the vital signs and proper urine output. Do not give any parenteral or oral nutrients for two to four weeks. Life can be sustained with proper fluids and Autoimmune urine therapy for 100 days without much ill effects.
6. Monitor all the vital signs similar like you monitor critically ill patients in intensive care. Treat all the complications with modern medications symptomatically. As you are feeding urine, the dose of the drugs if they are need, are reduced. I would avoid giving any drug unless it is absolutely indicated (i.e. life is threatened if not given).
7. Maintain proper ventilation. Do not give too much oxygen. Maintain blood oxygen levels of 100 mm Hg. Too much oxygen for long periods of time can be toxic to the lungs and inhibit the immune system. Oxygen saturation can be measured by a simple pulse oximeter.

8. Continue the therapy for 2-3 weeks or as long as the patient shows the signs of improvement. If the brain shows no activity as measured by EEG, evaluate the treatment.

How Does This therapy Cure?

This AUT and hyperthermia therapy is based on theory like any other discovery. The heat will kill many of rabies virus. They will come out in the urine in large quantities, partially denatured by heat. When these antigens and other substances in the urine are taken orally, stimulates the immune system as describe in chapter 1,7,8,9,10,11,12,13,18. Many of the explanation given for tuberculosis, AIDS, and leprosy also applies here. Rabies virus increases the level of quinolinic acid in the brain, a neurotoxic convulsant metabolite of tryptophan by 1000 fold or more as seen in other viral infections. Hyperthermia and AUT neutralizes this metabolite and the enzyme responsible for it. That is why this therapy has a chance of successes in rabies.

Anybody wanting to try this method on animal experimentation and/or rabies afflicted people, please call me at this number (404-496-1482/0809). I will be happy to guide this experimental therapy by phone and will be available to supervise the therapy. I need actual cases to test my theory. Please give me a chance to prove or disprove my thinking and rationale behind this treatment. If I thought for a movement that it is only a theory and has no chance of succeeding, I would not document in writing and risk my scientific carrier.

GIVE MY METHOD OF TREATMENT DESCRIBED IN THIS BOOK A CHANCE BEFORE YOU CRITICIZE

For most incurable diseases other than rabies, intubation, ventilation, paralyzing the patients, intensive care type therapy with various monitors may not be needed. All they need is hyperthermia and autoimmune urine therapy as described in this book. The treatment and monitoring must be tailored according to the condition of the patient, nature of the causative agents and the severity of the disease.

Leprosy and Tuberculosis: Hyperthermia, AUT, With or Without Drugs

There are about 10 millions leprosy patients and one million new cases are add every year all over the world. Leprosy like rabies is known from biblical days. Leprosy is caused by lepra bacillus. The patients have to take the drugs such as dapsone(a sulfone) for years or all their life. This long therapy has been shortened by addition of new antimicrobial agents. Millions of people in underdeveloped countries also suffer from tuberculosis. Like leprosy it is also caused by an acid fast tuberculosis bacillus. This is because of overcrowding, poor nutrition and lack of facilities to detect and treat early infection. These patients are treated using antibacterial drugs such as streptomycin, PAS, and INH.

All we need in these patients is moderate to severe hyperthermia combined with AUT with or without anti leprosy and anti tuberculosis drugs. I do believe that this combination of therapy will achieve a better and faster cure than conventional therapy. Patient may not have to take drugs for years as it is done now.

Hyperthermia and AUT probably cures or curtails leprosy and tuberculosis as described below.

1. Heat kills the bacteria.
2. The killed bacterial components come out in the urine.
3. When taken back orally stimulate the immune system.
4. Hyperthermia itself stimulates the immune system (see chapter 1).
5. Hyperthermia weakens the cell membrane of leprosy and tuberculosis bacteria and the membrane of the infected cells. The drugs will get into these bacteria and cells infected with these bacteria easily because of the changes created by hyperthermia. Because of the malfunctioning cell membrane, the drugs will not easily exits from the bacteria and cell infected with the bacteria. This results in higher concentration of the drug within the bacillus and the cells infected with these bacteria, ultimately resulting in their death.
6. There is a slow absorption of dead or weakened bacteria (virus in rabies and other viral diseases) and infected cells. This leads to the potentiation of host immune system (Chapter 1).

Many of the explanations given how hyperthermia and AUT works in chapter 1, 6,7,8,9,10,11,12,13,18 also apply here. Tuberculosis is also caused by an acid fast bacillus. It can also be treated with moderate hyperthermia and AUT with or without drugs. There are many reports of tuberculosis cure by AUT. Combining it with hyperthermia will enhance the effectiveness of the therapy. The details are described in Volume II on this subject.

I want leprologist and tuberculosis specialists try my method of treatment. If you don't want to combine with AUT, try hyperthermia and drugs. Results will be startling. The leprosy and tuberculosis patients do not need complicated monitoring like rabies patients during hyperthermia. They need not be intubated. All they need is sedation during hyperthermia.

Other Diseases that can be Treated with AUT and Hyperthermia

The list is endless and reads like a text book of medicine. I want to open a research institute to treat these diseases.

1. Any viral, bacterial, fungal, spirochetal, rickettsial, parasitic or any other kind of unknown microbial infections, poisonous bites.
2. Any acute or chronic diseases that does not respond to conventional methods of treatment or there is no therapy.
3. Autoimmune diseases.
4. All kinds of cancers.
5. Central and peripheral nervous system diseases.
6. Coronary artery and other blood vessel diseases.
7. Allergic conditions and associated diseases such as asthma, running nose and eyes etc.and all skin diseases.
8. Many metabolic diseases.
9. Some genetic diseases such as muscular dystrophy, sickle cell anemia etc. If it does not cure, it will at least hold in check, and prolong the life.
10. Cancer of the oesophagus, prostate, breast, bladder, rectum, peritoneal cavity, cervix, vagina etc.

CHAPTER 20

THE MIND, BODY, IMMUNE SYSTEM AND HEALING

Physiologically and pharmacologically, feelings are chemicals,
They can make you happy or sick,
They can cure or kill.

T. R. Shantha

Disease in man is never exactly the same as the same disease in an experimental animal, for in man the disease at once affects and is affected by what we call the emotional life.

Francis W. Peabody

May, he protect us both; May, we attain vigor together
May, we not cavil at each other, OM Shanthi, Shanthi, Shanthi (peace).

Katha Upanishad

As he thinks in his heart, so he is.

Proverbs 23:7

A sound mind in a sound body; if the former be glory of the latter, the latter is indispensable to the former.

Tryon Edward

The Power of Positive Thinking

There is increasing evidence to show that the mind does play an important role in healing. This has been shown in patients with cancer, chronic pain sufferers, asthma, and mental disorders, and many other incurable, chronic diseases. This is also true in AIDS patients. When a faith healer performs his healing ministry curing various diseases, it is your belief in the healing that healed you, not the faith healer. Dr. Richard B. Shakelle, Ph.D., of the University of Texas health Medical Center of Houston studied 2000 industrial employees for two decades. Those who scored highest on depression were more than likely to die of cancer than the rest of the group.

Just the power of positive thinking is not good enough. Support it by proper treatment plan. There is a possibility that the addiction and some mental disorders can be treated with hyperthermia in combination with autoimmune urine therapy. Those persons feeling a lack of control, helplessness, depression, difficulty in expressing negative emotions, missing self-satisfaction and who are excessively polite are called type "C" personality. They are worse when it comes to surviving chronic illnesses such as cancer and AIDS.

Psycho-Neuro-Immunology (PNI)

A person's mood, feelings, state of mind, behavior, attitude, and coping ability can affect the immune system. This science has been named psycho-neuro-immunology (PNI). In the book The Healer Within (Dutton), by Drs. Locke and Levy, explains PNI and its physiologic link between the brain, the nervous system and immune system. People under stress release a stress hormone called corticosteroid. This hormone depresses the immune system, including the action of macrophages and white blood cells. Such people do not cope well with stressful situations. The study also showed that sadness diminished the activity of lymphocyte natural killer cells (T8 lymphocyte). A study of healthy college students showed that those students who had many symptoms of depression had diminished tumor-killing ability in their white blood cells. There is evidence linking a "broken heart" to a damaged immune system. Months after a wife's death, a man can show a striking decline in white blood cell function. Hyperthermia and AUT therapy can effectively enhance the psycho-neuro-immune system.

Production of Healing Substances in the Brain

There is scientific evidence showing that the mind, body and immune system are bound together. We already know that certain substances produced by the brain transform thoughts and reactions into chemicals. These chemicals, in turn, affect the body positively or negatively. To put it in laymen's language, feelings are chemicals which make you happy or depressed, cure you or kill you. Cure by any means, whether through faith healers, visiting holy places, psychotherapy, religious healers, hypnotherapy, cult healers, quantum healing, drinking Ganges water, occurs because they fill the soul, heart and body with joy, hope, love and inner peace. This translates into a positive response from the body's immune system. It also increases the level of good chemicals (endorphins and other hormones), thereby resulting in a decrease in the disease and its symptoms or in a complete cure. These modes of therapy should be practiced along with standard medical care provided by experts. Even if positive thinking therapy does not heal you completely, it can prolong your life, reduce your symptoms and add quality.

Dr. Deepak Chopra claim that he has cured many cancers with sensory modulation by using music, touch, smell, meditation, massage and diet (Quantum Healing: Exploring the frontiers of mind-body Medicine, Bantam 1989). He calls it quantum healing, a atomic age word for this ancient Ayurvedic method. He thinks that mental technique used in Ayurveda, a 5000 year old system of medicine form India, allows us to go deep inside to contact the hidden prints of intelligence and change it. Meditation can trigger the mind to influence the body and cure the disease. This concept is not much different from the faith healing, prayer healing, psycho immune therapy, visualization therapy etc. I believe that the meditation combined with AUT and hyperthermia has better chace of curing a disease than just meditating.

Relaxation Response

One of the problems with physicians is that they are often trained to diagnose and treat only the physical disease. The human being is an emotional being and needs love, hope and joy in addition to physical needs. By loving patients and caring for them, physicians may help them take suffering with ease. We must teach them to learn loving and caring for themselves. By loving yourself, you do communicate with your inner self. Deeds, words, hearing, smelling, seeing, meditation, hypnotic trance, yoga, prayer, etc., all can help put us in touch with our inner self, that has been ignored in this materialistic world. This is called a relaxation response. The relaxed body consumes less oxygen, respiration slows down, the blood pressure drops, muscle tension is reduced, cholesterol is lowered, and the blood flow to the heart is increased. Relaxation therapy reduces the need for insulin in diabetics, ends asthmatic attacks, and reduces the pain in arthritic people. Relaxation, along with visualization therapy, enhances curative therapy. The body defenses become even stronger, according to Howard University Psychologist, Mary Jasnoski, PhD.

**Unconditional Love of Yourself and Others:
A trademark of Inner Joy and Peace**

Love for yourself and for others should be unconditional. Loving is not boring, it is forgiving. It diffuses all pent-up feelings of hostility to others. There is really nothing to forgive yourself for. This is one of the first steps you must take to attain the power of hope, love, joy, in the inner self and inner peace. Once you develop inner peace, your whole life changes. According to Dr. B. S. Siegel (Peace, Love and Healing, Harper and Row, 1989) the symptoms of inner peace are:

1. You do not act due to fears based on experience.
2. Do not worry, enjoy every minute of your life.
3. You will not judge other people and their actions, neither judge harshly yourself or condemn your actions, accept things as they are, do not try to manipulate others to make things happen, love the loved.
4. Do not get involved in conflicts.

5. You appreciate what is good in other people.
6. You have expression of joy though smiling and eye contact.

Death is not escapable and comes on its own terms. The aim in life is to live an enjoyable, long, and happy life. The aim in life is not to escape death or be preoccupied with it. It is not when you die, it is how you lived that matters. Do what you want, not what someone else tells you what to do. It is your life. Inner peace, inner self, inner bliss, inner joy are more important than anything you possess. The body and mind that feels better, functions better.

How you perceive your situation in relation to yourself and your self image has lot to do with the way you react. The journey of life is not a smooth like a shot in butter. Everybody has their own problems and needs. Mental health is as important as physical health. Everybody has stress. Stress makes people go. It is how one channels the stress--in good or bad directions--that makes or breaks an individual.

Avoid Things that Can Make You Unhappy and Sick

You can be unhappy and sick if you:

1. Pay no attention to your physical body, indulge in excess of food, drinking and sex. Stress yourself to the maximum without venting your reactions and have no sense of humor.
2. Develop low esteem of yourself. Treat your life as meaningless, messed up. Follow what other people want instead of doing what you really want to do, complain constantly, feel stuck, miserable, worry all the time and have no sense of humor.
3. Blame others and yourself all the time and do not express your opinion honestly.
4. Think often about bad events that could happen.
5. Cut off yourself from family, friends and relatives, quit working on the basis your life is worthless.
6. Visit multiple doctors without taking care of yourself, feel that you have an awful life or that you would rather be dead than alive.

Avoid all the above situations or any other situation that makes you sick, depressed, restless and bad.

How to Stay Well and Avoid Sickness

To get well, you are to reverse all negative things making you sick and keeping you sick. You have to explode a bomb made up of "Positive thinking, joy, hope, and love." It releases power to all parts of your body. It is your body; handle it delicately as you would nurture a baby. It needs close attention. Adopt the following guidelines to change your sickness and get better (Dr. B. S. Seigel, 1989).

1. Engage in activity that brings joy, fulfillment, and purpose. According to the famous mythologist and sociologist (late) Joseph Campbell, follow your inner bliss. That is, do what you want and what makes you the happiest, instead of what other people say you should do. That is the true meaning of inner bliss or inner peace.
2. Take care of your physical body by proper nutrition and exercise. Make commitment to good health.
3. Express your feelings. Release all negative emotions, resentment, fear, sadness, envy. Forgive and love yourself and others. Keep a sense of humor. Focus your attention on images of love, peace and joy. Avoid fearful events. Hold positive feelings. Strive for realistic goals.
4. Have joyful, loving, honest, relationships with your mate, immediate family members, friends, relatives, and working associates.
5. Get involved with deeds that contribute positively to your and your community.
6. Develop your own healing program based on the advise of experts in the field. Do not become a slave to someone else,s program.
7. Practice mild to moderate hyperthermia and AUT at home to enhance all your body functions and support your psychological needs even if you are n;ot sick.

As Rev. Robert Schuller put it, "failure has an ending, success has no ending." Take failure as a stepping stone for success. Learn from failure and move on with your life goals. You must have determination to get rid of the disease and nothing is going to stop it. Avoid all stressful situations. Learn to resolve problems, don't let them linger. Be in control of the situation. Do not respond to stressful situations with feelings of helplessness, hopelessness, depression and anxiety. Don't repress--express. I highly recommend that all people, including AIDS patients, watch Dr. Robert Schuller's program on Sunday from Garden Grove, California. Read his books, they support your religious beliefs, lift your psyche, boost your immune system, and produce healing chemicals.

Visualization Therapy (V.T.)

V.T. is very similar to the psycho-neuro-immune (PNI) therapy discussed before, except V.T. is more regimented. This therapy is based on the premise that the psychological forces in the innermost part of the mind can actually help the development and advancement of diseases (tumors, AIDS, heart attack). These forces can also be consciously activated to battle and conquer the diseases. According to Dr. O. Carl Simonton of the Cancer Counseling and Research Center in Dallas, Texas, he self-healed skin cancer over his nose in one year using V.T. (How to Fight Cancer and Win, 1988, page 179, by William L. Fischer). Cancer patients under his care practicing V.T. are said to live twice as long as others. I do not recommend the V.T. as primary method of treatment.

V.T. for AIDS and Other Incurable Diseases

There are many ways of practicing V.T in AIDS and other chronic diseases, including cancer. You draw a picture of the AIDS virus (or cancer if you have cancer) depicted a monster. You then show how the good cells such as clones of activated T and B lymphocytes and macrophages are fighting this monster and winning. The important points to remember about this therapy is that you can never lie to your subconscious mind. Do not say to yourself that you are fine when you are actually ill. Do not try to cover the truth from yourself, because your subconscious mind always knows the truth.

First, recognize and acknowledge that you have the AIDS virus infection (or any other disease) and then reject this virus disease.

Imagine that you are not fighting with good guys in your body. Imagine that the AIDS virus is the villain. The immune system cells are the good guys, that attack and kill the villains. While practicing autoimmune urine therapy, imagine the "water with life" permeating the body and sweeping the viruses out of the body to the dumping ground or ocean. The HIV are being eaten by fish without any ill effects to the fish. Imagine a picture, draw it on the paper, and keep it in your mind. You can imagine T and B lymphocytes as raiders on white horses with shining armor and swords attacking the virus. You can also imagine them as modern warriors with laser guns. They are searching and zapping the ugly AIDS viruses in the circulation and those hiding within the cells.

Yours is a seek and destroy mission. Imagine an elaborate scheme in your mind and execute it. Once you have a strong mental image, your subconscious mind will deliver these images. Select a quiet place where you can relax and concentrate on your visualization therapy (VT). Practice VT two times a day with each session lasting for fifteen to twenty minutes a day. Add a few additional minutes of VT at the end of the day. The time it takes to achieve success depends on your commitment. Your ability to persuade the subconscious to direct the internal forces to attack and conquer the aggressor (AIDS, cancer, arthritis, etc.). Though there is documentation of the benefits of VT claims, it is not recognized and universally accepted by many physicians and scientists. All we can say is that it can only help to boost the hyperthermia, autoimmune urine therapy in containing the HIV infection, AIDS and other diseases.

Practicing mild to moderate hyperthermia, autoimmune urine therapy, along with the practice of PNI, VT and any other form of psychotherapy--religious or nonreligious--will help you to conquer the disease. It will help you to lead a life filled with joy and inner bliss in spite of the disease. It will also help you to accept the given situation with grace. It will ward of all the fears that surround the disease. It will change your life and change your disease for the better.

Hyperthermia and AUT to improve the Brain Function to Boost Psychotherapy

Hyperthermia like meditation also increases the levels of endorphins which in turn reduces the pain in the body. There is good possibility that with hyperthermia, the brain will get rid of some of the atherosclerotic patches in the brain blood vessels and thus increase the brain circulation and function. Hyperthermia also rids many macromolecules in between the brain cells and other cells (glial cells) surrounding them. The macromolecule and amorphous material accumulate between the brain cell connections (synapses) which slows down brain impulse conduction. These substances are reduced by hyperthermia thus increasing the brain function. The glial cells become very active and remove some of the non functioning, unwanted material from the nerve cells, their surrounding, and their synapses. That is why I believe that patients with Alzheimer's disease can be helped if hyperthermia is combined with the autoimmune urine therapy.

These therapies will help to clean up the brain cells and their surroundings. The heat of hyperthermia and the turbulent circulatory changes associated with it will help to break the blood brain barrier, dislodge the amorphous and other toxic material in the nervous system and remove it from the brain. It also cleans the blood vessels. In AIDS the viral components affecting the brain function including quinolinic acid are denatured, neutralized and removed from the brain due to heat and turbulent blood flow. Many of the mental and nervous system symptoms of AIDS will be reduced or eliminated with practice of hyperthermia and AUT. I do believe that AUT and hyperthermia can be effective in all kind of chemical dependency (drugs, tobacco, alcohol and all other kinds of addictions).

CHAPTER 21

APPEAL FOR FUNDING TO OPEN A RESEARCH INSTITUTE TO STUDY AUTOIMMUNE URINE THERAPY AND HYPERTHERMIA

Ask and it will be given to you; seek and You will Find;
knock and the door will be opened to you.
Matthew 7:7

I am appealing for the funds to establish a research institute (Hyperthermia and Autoimmune Urine Therapy Institute - HAUTI) to study hyperthermia and autoimmune urine therapy on various viral and other microbial diseases and other acute and chronic curable and incurable diseases. The whole study on human volunteers will cost no more than a test missile fired in the Defence Department. I estimate that it will cost about 25 million dollars for a ten year study. A preliminary study costing about two to three millon dollars for one year will tell us whether we should continue with this project or not. I can convince hospitals to take up the study of hyperthermia and AUT. **I will not use the life threatening extracorporeal method to induce hyperthermia. Instead I will use the radiant heat or other methods which are safe and does not need a team of highly skilled anesthesiologists, surgeons and technicians.** The funds should be able to support my present income for the next 10 years so that I can devote all my energies to eradicate or control this disease. This project, if successful, can be extended to include leprosy, tuberculosis, cancer, cancer of the esophagus, Alzheimer's disease, leukemia, muscular dystrophy, rabies, multiple sclerosis, autoimmune diseases, and many other incurable diseases. I had set up a project for rabies treatment using the same guidelines. Due to lack of funds, I could not proceed with the project.

I need funds. Philanthropists, charitable organizations or governments agencies, American or any other country, please help me to undertake this project.

I will be happy to advise any individual patient with AIDS or with any other disease such as rabies, leprosy, tuberculosis, cancer, and many other diseases which there is no effective therapy, on a patient-to-doctor basis. I need to obtain from the patients that I will not be medicolegally liable for any unforseen complications arising out of this therapy. People can set up their own hyperthermia set up in their home to induce mild to moderate hyperthermia as described in chapter 1. I believe that I may have better than fifty fifty chance of succeeding in my treatment. All I need is funds to start this project. Thousands of children may not die of AIDS and other incurable diseases if they follow my therapy.

Autoimmune urine therapy and hyperthermia is simple, cost free, and harmless if proper guidelines are followed, and it can CURE OR CURTAIL DISEASES. Please help me, fund me, together we can conquer these menacing diseases.

For anyone or agency or government or charitable foundations etc. willing to fund the research project please contact:

T. R. Shantha, M.D., Ph.D.
1657 Kanawha Drive,
Stone Mountain, Georgia, USA. 30087
Phone number: (404) 496-0809

REFERENCES

The following is a partial list of references consulted during the preparation of this manuscript. Some references are cited in the text. JAMA=The Journal of American Medical Association.

AIDS: A guide for Survival, Houston Acad. of Medicine, 1987.

AIDS Weekly Surveillance Report. Centers for Disease Control; February 1, 1988.

Armstrong JW. The water of life. C. W. Daniel Co. LTD, London, 1944.

Allain JP, et al. Edited. Human Retroviruses and Diseases They Cause. Abbot Centennial Symposium, Published by Excerpta Medica, Princeton, NJ, May 1988.

American Foundation for AIDS Research (AmFAR), AIDS/HIV experimental Treatment directory, Vol. 2, May 1988.

Atlanta Journal and Constitution reports: AIDS Could Virtually Cripple Third World, Expert Says. March 28, 1987; Unapproved AIDS Drug Stirs Alarm. April 30, 1988; Virus, The Ultimate Parasite. Jan. 27, 1987.; Leper Colony, An Army Base Combats AIDS. March 5, 1989.

American Medical Association News: Soviet MD Relates HIV Infection Incident Involving 73 Children. Teens Seen As Next Group of New AIDS Cases. June 16, 1989.; MD With AIDS Suspended From Hospital. February, 1987.

Bolognnesi PD. Prospects for prevention of and early intervention against HIV. JAMA, 261, 3007-313, 1989.

Cleary et al. Compulsory Premarital Screening for the Human Immunodeficiency Virus. JAMA, October 2, 1987.

Cole HM, and Lundberg GD., Editors. AIDS: From the Beginning. Journal of the American Medical Association, 1986.

Creagh-Kirk et all. Survival Experience Among Patients With AIDS Receiving Zidovudine: Follow-up Of Patients in a Compassionate Plea Program. JAMA, November 25, 1988.

DeVita VT, Hellman S, and Rosenberg SA. AIDS: Etiology, Diagnosis, Treatment, and Prevention. W. B. Saunders, New York, 2nd. Ed., 1988.

Ebbesen P, Bigger RJ, Melby M. AIDS, A Basic Guide for Clinicians. W.B.Saunders Co, Phil. 1984.

Emory Cancer News. Immunotherapy Trial Targets Melanoma and Renal Cancer. February 1988.

FDA Drug Bulletin. Special AIDS Issue. September 1987.

Fischl MA., et al. Safety and Efficacy of Sulfamethoxazole and Trimethoprim Chemoprophylaxis for Pneumocystis carinii Pneumonia in AIDS. JAMA, February 26, 1988.

Friedland GH, and Klein RS., Transmission of Human Immunodeficiency Virus, New England J of Medicine, Oct. 29, 1987, Vol. 317, No. 18.

Gallo RC., The First Human Retrovirus. Scientific American, December 1986.

Gallo RC. The AIDS Virus. Scientific American, January 1987.

Gaspari et al. Dermatologic Changes Associated with Interleukin 2 Administration. JAMA, September 25, 1987.

Gostin LO. Public Health Strategies for Confronting AIDS. JAMA, March 17, 1989.

Groopman JE. Taking Care of AIDS Patients. The Internist, April 1987.

Guinan ME., and Hardy A, Epidemiology of AIDS in Women in the United States. JAMA, April 17, 1987.

Hahn et al. Prevalence of HIV Infection Among Intravenous Drug Users in USA. JAMA, May 12, 1989.

Hearst N, Hulley SB. Preventing the Heterosexual Spread of AIDS. JAMA April 22, 1988.

Jaroff, L. The Gene Hunt. Time, March 20, 1989.

Kessler HA, Blaauw B, et al. Diagnosis of HIV Infection in Seronegative Homosexuals Presenting With An Acute Viral Syndrome. JAMA, Sept. 4, 1987.

JAMA. Human Immunodeficiency Virus Infection in Transfusion Recipients and Their Family Members. April 10, 1987.

JAMA. Antibody to Human Immunodeficiency Virus in Female Prostitutes. April 17, 1987.

JAMA. Recommendations for Prevention of HIV Transmission in Health-Care Settings. September 18, 1987.

JAMA. Immunodeficiency Virus Slowly Yields Secrets. June 17, 1988.

JAMA. Passionate Kissing and Micro lesions of the Oral Mucosa: Possible Role in AIDS Transmission. Jan. 13, 1989.

JAMA. Cessation of Zidovudine Therapy May Lead to Increased Replication of HIV-1. February 10, 1989.

JAMA. Links Between Cocaine and Retroviral Infection. Jan. 27, 1989.

JAMA. Various Approaches to AIDS Vaccines Begin to 'Pierce the Armor of Virus. July 7, 1989.

JAMA. Epoetin Alfa Approved for Anemia Treatment; Aerosolized Pentamidine Approved for PCP Prophylaxis. July 14, 1989.

JAMA. Projection of AIDS morbidity and mortality in San Francisco, March. 16, 1990

Krasinski K, and Borkowsky. Measles and Measles Immunity in Children Infected with HIV. JAMA, May 5, 1989.

Lechtenberg R and Hollenberg J. AIDS in The Nervous System. JAMA, February 17, 1989.

Levy AJ, Human immunodeficiency virus and the pathogenesis of AIDS. JAMA, 261, 2997-3006, 1989

Newsweek. AIDS: A Bad Way to Die. March 23, 1987. A Perilous Double Love Life. July 13, 1987.

Okie S. Genes May Play Role in Contracting AIDS. The Washington Post, May 1987.

Patel RM. Manavamootra, swamootra, Kannada translation, Published by Sahitya Bhandara, Hubli, Karnataka State, India, 1965

Pekkanen J. AIDS: The Plague That Knows No Boundaries. Reader's Digest, June, 1987.

Rinaldi RC. HIV Blood Test Counseling: AMA Physician Guidelines. AMA, 1988.

Rosen S, Editor. AIDS and The Nervous System. JAMA, April 28, 1989.

Sande, MA, and Volberding PA. Edited. The Medical Management of AIDS, 2nd Ed. W. B. Saunders Co Phila., 1988.

Scientific American: What science knows about AIDS. Oct. 1988, p.41-134.

Seigel SB. Peace, love and healing, Harper and Row, 1989.

Selwyn PA. AIDS: What is Now Known. HP Publi. Co. NY, 1986.

Selwyn PA. et al. Knowledge of HIV Antibody Status and Decisions to Continue or Terminate Pregnancy Among Intravenous Drug Users. JAMA, June 23, 1989.

Stone A. Cancer Therapy Draws Interest of Entrepreneurs. The Atlanta Journal, September 14, 1987.

Stryker D. Treating AIDS Related Infections. Hospital physician, March 1989.

Ubell E. When A Life Is In Your Hands. Parade Magazine, The Atlanta Journal Edition, March 5, 1989.

Wilentz A. Putting AIDS to the Test. Time, March 2, 1987.

INDEX